WATER FITNESS DURING YOUR PREGNANCY

Jane Katz, EdD
City University of New York

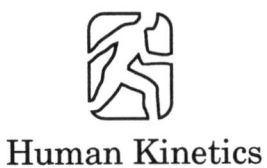

Human Kinetics

Library of Congress Cataloging-in-Publication Data

Katz, Jane.
  Water fitness during your pregnancy / Jane Katz.
    p.   cm.
  Includes index.
  ISBN 0-87322-495-7
  1. Pregnancy.   2. Aquatic exercises.   I. Title.
  RG558.7.K38   1995
  618.2'4--dc20   94-17659
                                                                   CIP

ISBN: 0-87322-495-7

Copyright © 1995 by Jane Katz

All rights reserved. Except for use in a review, the reproduction or utilization of this work in any form or by any electronic, mechanical, or other means, now known or hereafter invented, including xerography, photocopying, and recording, and in any information storage and retrieval system, is forbidden without the written permission of the publisher.

Notice: Permission to reproduce the following material is granted to persons who have purchased *Water Fitness During Your Pregnancy:* pages 214, 222-223. The reproduction of other parts of this book is expressly forbidden by the above copyright notice. Persons who have not purchased *Water Fitness During Your Pregnancy* may not reproduce any material.

Exercise and health are matters that vary from individual to individual. Readers should speak with their own doctors about their individual needs before starting any exercise program. This book is not intended as a substitute for the medical advice and supervision of your personal physician. Any application of the recommendations set forth in the following pages is at the reader's discretion and sole risk.

The W.E.T. Workout® is a registered trademark of Dr. Jane Katz.

Developmental Editor: Julia Anderson; **Assistant Editor**: Jacqueline Blakley; **Copyeditor**: Ginger Rodriguez; **Proofreader**: Myla Smith; **Indexer**: Theresa J. Schaefer; **Typesetter and Layout Artist**: Kathy Boudreau-Fuoss; **Text Designer**: Judy Henderson; **Cover Designer**: Jack Davis; **Illustrator**: Dianna Porter; **Printer**: United Graphics

Printed in the United States of America

10   9   8   7   6   5   4   3   2   1

Human Kinetics
P.O. Box 5076, Champaign, IL 61825-5076
1-800-747-4457

Canada: Human Kinetics, Box 24040, Windsor, ON N8Y 4Y9
1-800-465-7301 (in Canada only)

Europe: Human Kinetics, P.O. Box IW14, Leeds LS16 6TR, England
(44) 532 781708

Australia: Human Kinetics, 2 Ingrid Street, Clapham 5062, South Australia
(08) 371 3755

New Zealand: Human Kinetics, P.O. Box 105-231, Auckland 1
(09) 309 2259

Contents

Preface	vii
Acknowledgments	xi

Part I Preparing for a Healthy Pregnancy and Recovery — 1

Chapter 1 Why Take the Plunge? — 3

What Is Water Fitness?	3
How Water Exercise Benefits Pregnancy	5
Pros and Cons of Water Exercise	8

Chapter 2 Starting Properly and Getting Equipped — 13

Health and Safety Guidelines	13
General Workout Tips	15
Water Exercise Equipment	17

Part II Water Exercise Techniques: The W.E.T. Workout Program for Pregnancy — 23

Chapter 3 Warm-Up and Cool-Down Exercises — 25

Overhead Stretch	27
Sit and Kick	28
Feet Flex	29
Water Walk/Jog	30
Shoulder Shrug	31
Stand Tall	32

Pelvic Tilt	33
Water Kegel	34
Aqua Lunge	35
Effleurage	36

Chapter 4 Breathing Exercises — 37

Cleansing Breath	38
Breathe and Reach	39
Breathing With Head Circles	40
Breathe and Bob	41
Labor and Delivery Breathing Patterns	42

Chapter 5 Upper-Body Exercises — 45

Medley of Pulls	46
Arm Press	47
Arm Circle	49
Sport Swing	50
Hang 10	51
Sculling	52
Wall Push-Up	53
Kickboard Press	54

Chapter 6 Middle-Body Exercises — 55

Circle Spray	56
Hip Touch	57
Back Extension	58
Modified Sit-Up	60
Swing and Sway	61
Wall Knee Lift	62
Back Massage	63

Chapter 7 Lower-Body Exercises — 65

Flutter Kick	66
Bicycle Pedal	67
Leg Scissors	68
Calf Stretch	69
Wall Walk	70
Leg Lift	71
Leg Swirl	72
Double Leg Circle	73

Chapter 8 Total-Body Exercises — 75

Arm and Leg Reach	76
Pendulum Body Swing	77
Treading	78

Posture Check	80
Deep-Water Jog	81

Part III Swim Strokes — 83

Chapter 9 Crawl Stroke — 85

The Stroke	85
Crawl Stroke Refinements	88
Push-Off	89
Turn	90
Rhythmic Breathing	93
Catch-Up Arm Stroke	94

Chapter 10 Breaststroke — 95

The Stroke	95
Push-Off	98
Turn	98
Breaststroke Arm Pull	99
Frog Kick	100

Chapter 11 Backstroke — 103

Sculling	103
Elementary Backstroke	105
Windmill Backstroke	106
Push-Off	108
Turn	110
Scull and Hug	113
Back Flutter Kick	114

Chapter 12 Sidestroke — 115

The Stroke	115
Push-Off	118
Turns	118
Under and Over	120
Apple Picking	122

Part IV Your Water Fitness Program — 123

Chapter 13 First-Trimester Workouts — 129

Month 2	130
Month 3	134

Chapter 14 Second-Trimester Workouts — 141

Month 4	141
Month 5	146
Month 6	151

Chapter 15 Third-Trimester Workouts — 157
Month 7 — 158
Month 8 — 164
Month 9 — 169

Part V Postpartum Water Fitness Program — 175

Chapter 16 Getting Back in Shape — 177
Postpartum Water Exercise Guidelines — 177
Water Ballet Exercises — 178
Butterfly Stroke — 186
Postpartum Workouts — 193

Chapter 17 Expanding Your Water Exercise Program — 213
Masters Swimming — 213
Synchronized Swimming — 215
Water Play With Your Newborn — 215
Family Swimming Programs — 217

Appendix — 221
Index — 225
About the Author — 233

Preface

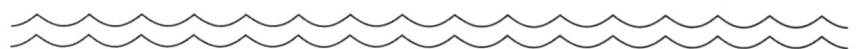

Some things never change. One of these is the natural wonder of pregnancy. From beginning to end, the course of pregnancy is the same today as it was centuries ago. Another continuing wonder is water, long used for growth, nourishment, cleansing, and refreshment. Its natural properties relax us, its buoyancy supports us. We enjoy the "weightless" feeling of being in water.

But other things have changed. One of these is the greater awareness of the importance of fitness. As medical knowledge has increased, we have learned that taking responsibility for one's own health is the smart thing to do. We have begun to evaluate what we eat and to make healthier lifestyle choices, adopting good nutrition and aerobic exercise as part of our lives.

As North American health standards have risen and more information has been made available on the correlation between healthy mothers and healthy babies, fitness during pregnancy has become a concern to more women. Exercise during pregnancy has become acceptable both to doctors and to women in general.

Swimming has long been a familiar activity, both for pleasure and for health, but exercise done in the water is newer and increasingly popular. This aerobic activity is ideal for pregnant women, and can be inexpensive. You can enjoy the refreshing and relaxing feeling of water while you exercise, which you will welcome even more as your body expands.

Water fitness (swimming and water exercise) involves a minimum of physical stress, with no pounding. The buoyancy of the water gives you support so you can exercise with more ease. You can have longer, better fitness sessions and can get and stay in shape with less fatigue.

Water Fitness During Your Pregnancy gives guidelines for a safe, effective program of water exercise and swimming. This book will help you enjoy your pregnancy and prepare you for the birth process by teaching you how to stretch, tone, and strengthen your body—gently—through water exercise and swimming. Although no one can guarantee you a painless childbirth, following this program can give you the advantage of entering motherhood knowing that you have made the effort to be in optimum physical condition and have prepared yourself for an excellent recovery and return to fitness (and figure)!

The water workouts progress through each trimester. Because each pregnancy is unique, I'll guide you through choosing your own water fitness program based on your skill level, your energy level ("How do I feel?"), and other personal considerations. For example, if you are a new swimmer, you can begin water exercise immediately with an exercise like water walking. If you are a seasoned swimmer who wants to avoid swimming laps in a congested pool, water exercise is a great alternative.

Water Fitness During Your Pregnancy will help you use whatever water fitness skills you have to get your body ready for a comfortable pregnancy and a prepared delivery. Even if you don't swim "yet," you can enjoy the benefits of a water workout during your pregnancy.

Ideally, a woman begins her pregnancy in the best possible physical condition. If you are fit this book will help you stay fit. However, if you are not in good physical condition, *Water Fitness During Your Pregnancy* will help you improve your fitness and comfort levels during pregnancy and to prepare for labor and delivery.

This guide will not teach you to swim. Rather, it presents water exercises, reviews swim stroke fundamentals, and suggests appropriate exercises for each trimester. It incorporates safety considerations throughout the text and answers questions you may be thinking about, but don't know where to ask.

Part I of *Water Fitness During Your Pregnancy* explains how exercising, particularly swimming, can help you through and after your pregnancy. It discusses how and why exercising in the water during your pregnancy can promote strength, flexibility, cardiorespiratory conditioning, and just plain comfort. Part I also highlights starting properly, gearing up appropriately, and warming up.

Part II introduces Water Exercise Techniques (WET) to prepare each body area for pregnancy and delivery. These WETs include individual exercises for warm-up and cool-down, breathing, upper body, middle body, lower body, and total body. Every exercise is thoroughly described and illustrated, so you'll know how to perform them correctly.

The swimming program in Part III reviews the mechanics of the crawl stroke, breaststroke, backstroke, and sidestroke and explains how to modify each stroke during pregnancy. Part III also discusses appropriate push-offs and turns.

Part IV focuses on formulating your own water fitness program for each trimester. This part helps you choose an appropriate workout given your body's month-by-month changes, whether you are swimming laps, exercising in the water, or doing some of both.

The postpartum program in Part V helps you get back into shape after delivery. This program provides a recovery workout and introduces other water fitness skills including synchronized swimming, butterfly, and Masters swimming. Part V also expands your water fitness fun with tips for family swimming and for introducing your baby to the water. It includes sources of information about swimming so you can find out where and how to enjoy the water with your family.

Here is my personal invitation to add water to the wonders of your childbearing time. I hope and trust that *Water Fitness During Your Pregnancy* will help you to be stronger, healthier, and more ready to begin life with your new baby. So take the plunge—the water's waiting for you!

ACKNOWLEDGMENTS

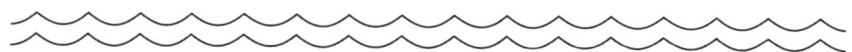

I'd like to give special thanks to:

My parents, Dorothea and Leon, who introduced me to the wonders of the water at an early age.

My sisters, Elaine Kuperberg and June Guzman, who swam through and after their pregnancies, and their children, Stephen, Jason, and Justin.

My brother Paul, for sharing his expertise in swimming; his wife Arden, and their son Austen.

Herbert L. Erlanger, MD, Attending Anesthesiologist, New York Hospital-Cornell Medical Center, for his sharing, caring, and support.

Desider J. Rothe, Clinical Associate Professor of Obstetrics and Gynecology, New York Hospital-Cornell Medical Center.

Elaine Fincham, MA, Recreation Therapist, Maryland/General, Pratt-Shepherd Hospital, and Oak View Treatment Center, MD; Constance M. Gold, RN, MA, ASPO Lamaze Childbirth Specialist, Bronx, NY; Howard Chislett, EdD, Columbia University; and Helen B. Pennoyer, MSW, ASPO Prepared Childbirth Instructor, New York, NY, for their valuable input and assistance.

Zvi Barak, PhD; Farida Gadalla, MD; Stephen B. Kurtin, MD; Janet Mines, RPT; Willibald Nagler, MD; and Thomas Verny, MD, for their advice and comments.

To the entire staff at Human Kinetics, especially the "team" who worked so hard on this book: Ted Miller, acquisitions editor; Julia Anderson, developmental editor; Jacqueline Blakley, assistant editor; Kathy Boudreau-Fuoss, typesetter and layout artist; and Dianna Porter, illustrator.

Anne Goldstein, for helping to type the manuscript.

To Julie See, President of the Aquatic Exercise Association, for her support and encouragement.

Angela Buchanan, Wendy Boglioli, Jill Clayburgh, Joyce Bloom, Barbara Crossen, Joan Grubbe, Cindy Kurtin, Linda Lebsack, Gaby Lehrer, Marcy Miller, Louise Dembeck-Neeman, Jan Stickley, Joy Taylor, Rosemary Young, my pregnant swimmers at Bronx Community College and John Jay College of Criminal Justice, and many fitness and Masters swimmers, for sharing their swimming experiences during and after their pregnancies.

Carole Andrews, Susan Caton, Cindy Clevenger, Pat Earle, Margaret Forbes, Mary Ann Jasien, Anita Karabelas, Millie Leinweber, Suzanne Michelle, Carol Miller, Jon S. Netts, the American National Red Cross, Marcellino Rodriguez, Michael Ross, PhD, Susan Schaefer, Tony Stafferi, Nick Stringas, Holly Turner, Lorraine Martinelli, and Sue Bessette for all their help.

Teri Kateri DePuy and Loys Green of the Health Promotion Department of the New York City YWCA for their special help. And to Patricia Spengel-Bauman, Nancy Meyer, and their fellow swimmers. And Joan Craffey.

Linda Ehrlich, RN, MS (Department of Anesthesia, Montifiore Hospital, Bronx, New York); Gunnel Greenfield, RN, (Infection Control Research, Beth Israel Medical Center, New York City); and to Pat Berland and Geraldine Griffen, RN, also of New York City.

Donna Glass, RN (Nurse Obstetrics, Beth Israel Medical Center, New York City) for her time and special help.

The Birthing Center of the Beth Israel Medical Center, Newark, New Jersey, with special thanks to Donna Russo, and to the Morristown General Hospital Prenatal Health Department, New Jersey.

And to the many women and children who inspired me and swam with me. Many thanks to you all, and especially to E.K.K.

To all parents, who bring life into the world, and especially to my parents, Dorothea and Leon, who introduced their children and many others to the wonders of the water. And to Adria Lynn.

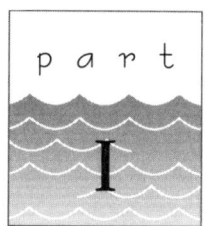

part I

PREPARING FOR A HEALTHY PREGNANCY AND RECOVERY

Congratulations! In a few months you'll become a new mother! Pregnancy is a special time of your life, not a debilitating condition. Most obstetricians now believe that a woman who does some type of physical conditioning during her pregnancy may be less likely to have difficulty during labor and childbirth, and they encourage their patients to be physically active. Even women who have not been physically active prior to pregnancy now are being encouraged to begin sensible programs of physical conditioning as soon as possible, though more slowly than women who are already fit. Pregnancy is no time to begin a vigorous exercise program if you have not already been exercising at that level. It is fine, however, to begin slowly and build to a moderate level.

This first part of the book focuses on background information about water, fitness, and pregnancy and how you can combine them safely and practically. Chapter 1, "Why Take the Plunge?" details how water and fitness together can help you have the best pregnancy possible. Chapter 2, "Starting Properly and Getting Equipped," gives the specifics of using water during pregnancy to improve your fitness level and prepare you for childbirth.

As with any fitness program during pregnancy, you should not begin this program without the approval of your doctor, and your doctor should be kept advised of your activity throughout your pregnancy.

Why Take the Plunge?

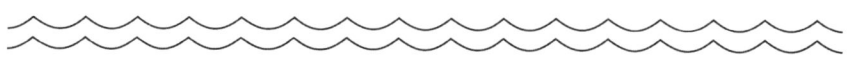

Most obstetricians now encourage their patients to engage in some form of physical conditioning, believing that a woman whose body is in good physical condition may be less likely to have difficulty during labor and childbirth. Women who have not been physically active prior to pregnancy now are being encouraged to begin programs of physical conditioning as soon as possible.

Appropriate exercise improves your cardiorespiratory fitness, promoting a strong heart and lungs, efficient circulation, and efficient oxygen utilization, all of which are important components for a comfortable pregnancy and an ideal labor and delivery. A healthy cardiovascular system is important for your baby because blood must be efficiently transported from your body to the placenta, which provides your baby with oxygen and nourishment. An improved fitness level is an asset throughout pregnancy because it helps minimize the fatigue most women experience.

Another reason to exercise during pregnancy is to strengthen and tone muscles you will use during the birth process. When you complete your pregnancy in good condition you are better prepared for the physical demands of childbirth (they don't call it "labor" for no reason!).

What Is Water Fitness?

You might define *water* as the colorless, transparent liquid occurring on earth as rivers, lakes, oceans, and so forth, and falling from the clouds as rain. Similarly, you could define *fitness* in terms of the condition of being fit, suitability, appropriateness, and healthiness. But what happens when you combine these two? You get *water fitness*, an enjoyable, low-impact way to better health. Water fitness includes swimming and exercising in both shallow and deep water.

For years, people have been swimming laps for fitness. The aerobic, muscular, and psychological benefits of swimming laps are well known. But although the number of lap and fitness swimmers increased during the last two decades, 50% of Americans either had never learned to swim, had had a bad experience in or near the water and were afraid to swim, or did not swim well enough to use swimming for aerobic conditioning.

As the exercise boom of the 1970s and '80s progressed, a growing need for low-impact fitness choices became obvious. Injuries associated with high-impact exercise called for a fitness activity that would combine stretching, aerobic conditioning, strength training, and flexibility without risk to joints or limbs.

Water exercise was the answer. Many people, especially senior citizens, began to devise their own workouts by transferring land-based exercises to the water. Water exercise classes, at first called *hydro-calisthenics* or *hydro-slimnastics*, began to appear.

Water exercise can now be described as a program of land-based movements *adapted* to the water, done in a vertical position (as opposed to swimming, which is done in a horizontal position). Water has different properties than air and the exercises are done in a different way than on land. Now "aquarobics" or "aquacise" classes are standard at YMCAs and YWCAs, community pools, and health clubs throughout the country. Approximately 5 million people in the United States participate in some form of water exercise.

Water exercise workouts can include shallow-water and deep-water exercises. Shallow-water exercises, done in waist-, and chest-, or shoulder-deep water, are usually dry-land strengthening or stretching exercises adapted to take advantage of the special properties of water.

Deep-water exercises include walking, jogging, or variations such as cross-country skiing. Many deep-water runners are land runners who are in the pool because they want to keep moving while recovering from an injury. Other runners began deep-water running as part of rehabilitation and continue it in addition to their restored running programs. Deep-water running attracts a wide range of participants because it allows marathoners, triathletes, and cross-trainers to maintain their aerobic conditioning and specificity of training while preventing overuse injury. Deep-water running is an appropriate exercise for arthritis patients, who can move more freely in the water. Some people exercise in deep water simply to enjoy a pleasant, effective way to keep in shape.

How Water Exercise Benefits Pregnancy

If you're expecting your first baby the changes happening in your body are of great interest to you, and you probably have been reading avidly all about pregnancy. So here is an overview of the anatomy of your pregnancy and how water exercise can help you during your pregnancy and delivery.

The most significant change in your body during pregnancy is the size of your uterus. Your uterus is comprised of three layers of muscle, each playing a specific role in labor and in delivery. The uterus increases in strength and thickness as pregnancy progresses.

Because your uterus changes dramatically in both size and shape, it requires other muscles to maintain it in its proper position. Giant elastic bands known as the *broad ligaments* keep your uterus safely suspended in the middle of your pelvis. Surrounding your uterus are abdominal and pelvic floor muscles that also provide support and are part of the labor and delivery process. Good abdominal muscle tone, which is developed by water exercise, improves this support and will also help maintain the function of your intestines and other organs as they are displaced by your growing uterus.

As your pregnancy progresses, your weight increases, and there is a change in your center of gravity (the theoretical point in space where all your weight, for practical purposes, is located). Strong back and abdominal muscles can better accommodate this change, lessening the stress on your back, hips, and thighs. Also, during your pregnancy your breasts become larger and heavier as they prepare milk. The right exercises will strengthen the chest muscles that help support your breasts.

Surrounding your uterus is a bone structure known as the *pelvic girdle*, which helps position your uterus and acts as the "funnel" through which the baby travels during a vaginal birth. Good pelvic-muscle tone helps maintain the position of your pelvic girdle in relation to the rest of your body. During labor and delivery, relaxing your pelvic muscles will facilitate the baby's passage through the birth canal. By exercising these muscles in advance, you will have better control of them during the birth process. Also helpful for labor are strong abdominal and pelvic floor muscles. And if you have a Cesarean section birth, abdominal muscles that have been exercised may speed the healing process and make it more comfortable.

For every change occurring in your body during pregnancy, water exercise and swimming can help your body adapt to carrying your baby and alleviate common discomforts, while preparing your muscles for childbirth. For example, some water exercises specifically strengthen the pelvic girdle and pelvic floor muscles. And in the water you can swim or exercise to strengthen your abdomen, back, and shoulders to help carry your weight more easily and maintain good posture, which is important to a comfortable pregnancy. This can be the relief from back discomfort that mothers-to-be look for. Swimming and certain water exercises strengthen chest muscles to better support your breasts as they enlarge, helping to maintain your figure. You can prepare your leg muscles for labor and delivery and help minimize postpartum urinary difficulties through water exercises for your hips and thighs.

Another less obvious change in your body during pregnancy is your blood supply: it will increase 25% to 50%. Your heart may even beat a little faster than it did before pregnancy, imposing additional demands on it, which are normal. A regular water fitness program will equip your heart and circulatory systems to handle these demands with greater ease. A healthy system is important because blood must be transported from your body to the placenta, which provides the baby with oxygen and nourishment. Improved cardiovascular efficiency may help minimize swelling in your extremities, as well as help prevent varicose veins and hemorrhoids, which are more common during pregnancy. Improved fitness helps reduce the fatigue most women experience during pregnancy and will be an asset in the event that your child is born by Cesarean section.

Water fitness can also help reduce your blood pressure. Just being in the water causes your body to naturally rid itself of excess water and salt. These are often the cause of water retention which can result in edema and discomfort as well as potentially dangerous high blood pressure. Reducing water and salt in your body may also alleviate the stiffness caused by water retention that some women experience at the ankles and wrists.

Swimming and water exercise are cool, pleasant ways to keep your exercise program going without the risk of overheating. Swimming, because it is done in a horizontal position, eases the pressure of the uterus on the diaphragm, making your breathing more comfortable while you swim. It also facilitates blood flow by making it easier for the heart to pump blood throughout your body. During both swimming and water exercise, the support provided by the water helps to relieve the weight of your uterus on your bladder and pelvic organs.

Swimming and water exercise work along with your body's natural adaptations in preparation for your baby's birth. Toward the end of pregnancy, the body's connective tissue loosens up (this is the conspicuous pregnant "waddle"). Water exercise and swimming work along with this change by improving joint flexibility. There are water exercises to stretch pelvic and thigh muscles for the birth and to strengthen pelvic girdle muscles for an optimal recovery.

Water exercise can offer your legs some relief from discomfort because it requires you to put little or no weight on your feet as you exercise. And exercising in water can help reduce the possibility of developing varicose veins, which result from the extra demands on the circulatory system.

When you are pregnant, your blood volume increases, requiring your arteries and veins to handle more blood. In addition, the valves in the veins in your legs have to work against the pressure of the added weight of your abdomen. Under these stresses the valves can become less effective in returning blood to your heart and lungs so the veins become dilated, visible, and sometimes quite uncomfortable. An exercise program of swimming, water exercise, or both improves your circulatory system, and the buoyancy of the water can help relieve the demands on your legs and veins. Easing the discomfort of varicose veins is especially helpful for those mothers-to-be who are predisposed by genetic, weight, or other factors to varicose veins.

This brings us to weight control. Swimming and water exercise are wonderful ways to control your weight. Because you can continue being active throughout your pregnancy, it is easier to keep your weight gain to "baby only" amounts (baby, placenta, and amniotic fluid). This provides you with a more comfortable pregnancy and makes it easier to regain your original figure after delivery.

You'll find that water exercise and swimming are good for your mind as well as for your body. Water is a sensuous medium. Immersed in it, you seem to defy gravity. Most mothers-to-be who exercise in water appreciate the way it suspends them, especially during the last part of their pregnancy.

Water and Childbirth

Ideas to promote well-being in pregnancy and to make childbirth less traumatic have emerged throughout history. After World War II, Western health care providers began to experiment with natural childbirthing techniques in response to what many doctors and mothers felt was the over-intervention of the medical sphere in the birth process. Not only that, but the growing knowledge of the dangers of drugs led to interest in natural childbirth. Mothers who chose natural childbirth discovered a number of advantages. One was that they generally had a lower incidence of certain problems during labor. Also, they appreciated the opportunity to be alert enough to participate in the births of their babies.

In the 1950s, the French obstetrician Frederick Leboyer developed the childbirth technique of "birth without violence," which eases the transition of the newborn from the womb to the world. One technique the Leboyer method uses is to massage the newborn in lukewarm water immediately following delivery. The best-known labor technique, however, is based on the work of Dr. Fernand Lamaze (*Psychoprophylaxis in Childbirth*, 1951). Since the 1970s the Lamaze method has been the most popular prepared childbirth technique in the United States. It is an adaptation of two schools of thought. The first, based on the Pavlovian theory of the conditioned response, holds that when a woman is in labor, she will be able to exercise control over her body during a contraction. The second school of thought is the "fear-tension-pain" theory of the English doctor Grantly Dick-Read. Dr. Dick-Read's work, published in 1933, maintained that the more a woman is educated and informed about childbirth, the less she will fear the unknown during the impending labor and delivery. Less fear means less tension, and less tension means less pain. The Lamaze method simply adopted these theories and added some sound physiological principles for the various stages of labor. The relaxation techniques and exercises used to prepare for childbirth can be practiced in the water, which assists relaxation.

Since the 1980s other prepared childbirth techniques have come into use, including the Bradley method of husband-coached childbirth, which is popular in the western United States. Like the Lamaze method, the Bradley method trains the mother-to-be to take an active part in delivery. It is important to note that both methods educate you in the childbirth process and teach you to *manage* the childbirth contractions. They by no means promise you a pain-free delivery.

Another technique that is growing in popularity is water birth. The Russians first successfully experimented with delivering babies in water. Closer to home, the state-of-the-art birthing center at the Beth Israel Hospital Center in Newark, New Jersey, has been providing for water births since 1990. The unique feature of this birthing center is the large tub (5 feet by 8 feet by 2 feet) mothers can use during labor. If a woman chooses to give birth in the water, she will be fully informed of the differences between delivery in the water and out of water and will be given instructions for a water birth. Once the actual delivery begins, she must either stay in the tub or choose a bed birth. Husbands can remain with their wives in the tub up to the time of the delivery.

There is a strong possibility that you are considering using one of these techniques to deliver the baby you're expecting. If so, you'll find that this water fitness program relates to your prepared childbirth classes. The Lamaze method emphasizes breathing techniques, so if you have been preparing for the birth through water exercise and swimming, you optimize your chances of a more comfortable labor and delivery. And a mother-to-be who has been trained to identify her abdominal, pelvic, and uterine muscles is better prepared for the delivery.

Pros and Cons of Water Exercise

If you have been an active person up to now, you already know the benefits of exercise: vitality, strength, flexibility, weight control, and stress reduction. It is exciting to know that you can continue to enjoy these benefits safely during pregnancy with a water exercise and swimming program.

The Pros

Swimming and water exercise are unique among fitness activities because they don't place stress and strain on your joints or muscles. This big plus comes from the buoyancy of the water, which gives you support as you exercise and reduces the amount of perceived exertion for a given activity. This means you can exercise longer and more intensely. For example, in neck-deep water, your apparent body weight is one tenth of what it is on land. So if you weigh 120 pounds on land, you'll feel like you weigh 12 pounds in water. You'll probably really appreciate the "weightless" feeling of exercising in water as your body expands. In practical terms, you'll be more likely to complete your workouts because the water keeps you cool and comfortable. You can maintain optimal fitness with less fatigue. Another plus is that the water is soothing and relaxing.

Working out in water enables the pregnant woman to continue exercising as the baby grows. Women who have been exercising prior to pregnancy eventually need to make adaptations to their fitness programs. Early pregnancy discomforts such as nausea and fatigue, as well as the dangers of overheating in warm weather, can limit activity on dry land. The natural increase in joint looseness that develops during pregnancy may reduce gross motor skills and increase the possibility of back, hip, knee, and ankle injuries. For example, if you have been enjoying tennis or volleyball, your reduced agility could cause falls. Runners will have to cut down on distance, especially during warm weather. During the second

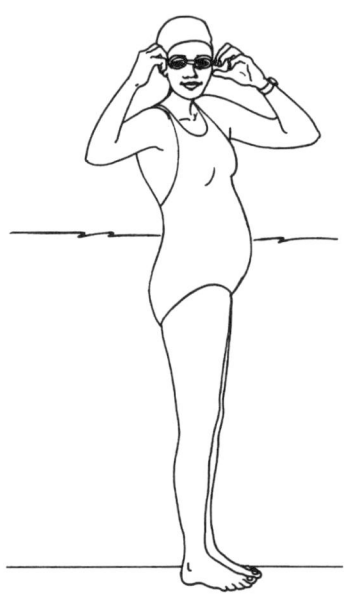

and third trimesters, your expanding abdomen changes your center of gravity, so skiing, cycling, and roller-blading become risky—just at the time when avoiding accidents is especially important. Lower-body edema (swelling) makes some sports inadvisable or just plain uncomfortable.

Workouts in water, whether water exercise, lap swimming, or a combination of both, are free from most of these risks. You can keep your muscles stretched and toned, maintain your cardiorespiratory fitness, and get cool, comfortable, and relaxed, all at the same time.

Swimming also helps control weight. A mother-to-be gains from 20 to 30 pounds during a normal pregnancy. An appropriate diet during your pregnancy is very important, both to protect your health and to assure proper prenatal development. Eating less to lose weight is generally not recommended for pregnant women. Swimming and water exercise can help keep off excess pounds during your pregnancy without dieting. In general, your pregnancy will be easier and more comfortable if you neither carry excess fat nor feel that you have to deprive yourself every time you sit down to eat.

The Cons

Past generations thought that exercise would harm a woman's reproductive organs and women's health in general. It was commonly believed that exercise during pregnancy would be dangerous to the unborn child and that moderate movement or bending during a normal pregnancy would harm the child. We know now that the uterus is a very well protected organ, guarded by strong ligaments and surrounded by pelvic bone. The unborn child is well protected from injury by the abdominal wall and the strong uterine muscle as well as by the amniotic fluid and sac.

There is ample evidence to indicate that exercising is beneficial rather than harmful for the pregnant woman, and does not harm the unborn baby either. So are there any "cons"?

No, not exactly. There are, however, considerations you may not have thought twice about before you became pregnant that assure the *safety* of you and your baby.

First, your water fitness environment must be clean, safe, and convenient. The pool and water should not appear dirty—a clean pool is a safe pool, but a pool with "ring around the collar" is one you should avoid. Moreover, if the locker room floor isn't kept clean, wear water shoes or nonskid sandals to avoid skin infection.

Think about "crowd control"—the number of people in the pool. Even if you are a seasoned swimmer experienced in sharing lanes with other swimmers, be sure you won't inadvertently be hit or kicked. If there are too many people in the pool, come back later when it is less crowded. Or, if possible, find a quiet corner for water exercise. There may be a deep end of the pool without a diving board in use that is less busy where you can do a deep-water workout. If you are fitting your swim into a busy schedule, check for other time blocks when you can exercise safely or look for other pools that fit more conveniently into your schedule.

The water temperature should be about 82 to 84 °F (28 °C). Temperature is important so you won't be cold and uncomfortable or take the risk of overheating.

It is very important to avoid overheating. Cardiorespiratory changes during pregnancy reduce your adaptability to heat stress. You run an increased risk of heat injury when you are exposed to high temperatures such as with vigorous exercise in hot weather, a Jacuzzi bath, a steam room, or sauna. In addition, *your baby doesn't have an air-conditioning system*; the fetus has no means of dissipating heat. Being overheated interferes with the baby's development, especially in early pregnancy. Therefore you should not use a Jacuzzi (hot tub), steam room, or sauna while you are pregnant, and you should avoid exercising in very warm weather. If you live in a warm climate and exercise outdoors, schedule your swim to avoid the strongest sun; swim early in the morning or later in the afternoon.

Naturally, your water fitness program should be adapted to fit the stage of your pregnancy. This book, together with your doctor's guidance, will show you how to adjust your swimming and water exercise program to meet your personal needs. So take the plunge and enjoy your pregnancy!

> **The water fitness program outlined in this book is suitable for all mothers-to-be, provided they have obtained their doctors' approval. You should not begin this program without the approval of your doctor, and your doctor should be kept advised of your activity throughout your pregnancy.**

chapter 2

STARTING PROPERLY AND GETTING EQUIPPED

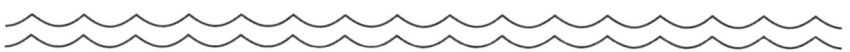

Water fitness and pregnancy are a great match! With a bit of preparation and some basic common sense you can be on your way to a healthful and relaxing workout that benefits both you and your baby. Here are some general considerations for starting your water fitness program properly.

A pleasant water fitness workout has to start in a pleasant pool. Find an aquatic facility in a reasonably convenient location with hours that are convenient for your schedule. The facility should be quiet, clean, and safe and offer ample locker area, preferably with sitting space. If the pool or changing facilities don't look clean, don't swim there until the problem is corrected. (The squeaky wheel gets the grease—speak up to the pool manager.) The water in the pool should ideally be 80 °F. Avoid a pool that's too cold—you're likely to get uncomfortable and possibly become discouraged. And avoid a pool that is too hot—that is a real safety hazard, especially at the beginning and end of your pregnancy. If a pool is very crowded, it is safer to swim at a less popular time.

Once you're there, don't overdo it. You don't feel the sweat and strain of exercise in the water, so you may not notice how strenuously you are moving. Be aware of how much you are doing in relation to your own fitness level, and pace your workouts. Be sure your fitness program is progressing gradually. This is not the time to become Wonder Woman (or Super Mom) overnight. If at any time you feel a strain, stop; if any discomfort persists, check with your doctor.

Health and Safety Guidelines

Then there are matters of safety. Of course, you will want to do everything you can to avoid health problems for you and your baby—this is one area where you should *never* cut corners!

First, follow your physician's recommendations regarding physical activity. Don't take chances with your health or the health of your baby. Do not begin this or any exercise program without the approval of your physician or childbirth professional. If you ever experience pain or bleeding, stop exercising and see your doctor.

It is very important to avoid overheating. Even if you think you *might* be pregnant, do not use a jacuzzi or sauna. Your body's "air-conditioning" system is less efficient during your pregnancy, and your baby does not have such a system at all. The baby depends on you to dissipate heat. So your baby's health is at stake.

Because of the dangers of overheating you must play it safe in the sun. If you are exercising outdoors, wear sunscreen and perhaps a sunhat or visor, and be careful not to overheat. Exercise itself heats up the body, so if it's a hot day and the water is warm, you might have to limit the energetic part of your workout. Or you can schedule your workout for the early morning or later in the afternoon, when the air is cooler.

Another danger of exposure to the sun is a condition called *chloasma* or *melasma* (sometimes called the "mask of pregnancy"). This is an excess of pigmentation on the upper lips, cheeks, and forehead that can develop during pregnancy because of elevated hormone levels. Keep in mind that water reflects and diffuses sunlight, so that even a short period of time at the beach or outdoor pool exposes you to a high level of the sun's ultraviolet rays without your being aware of it. If you must be out, use a sunscreen with the highest possible sun protection factor (SPF), and wear a protective hat or sun visor.

Because pregnancy-related hormonal changes affect some women's mucous membranes, increasing mucous secretion, they feel as if they have colds throughout their pregnancies. You may be one of these women. This condition should not prevent you from swimming during your pregnancy; in fact, swimming may help you feel better.

The chlorine in the pool will not adversely affect your health or cause any ill effects to your unborn child. Proper use of chlorine keeps the pool free of bacteria and algae and helps keep the water clear.

You can offset some of the effects of chlorine, however. Use goggles to protect your eyes from possible chlorine irritation. Shower after you swim to remove chlorinated water. Follow your shower with application of a moisturizing lotion to replace natural skin oils removed by the pool water. Be sure to clean and dry your feet carefully to keep them healthy and avoid possible infection.

If you have been doing the butterfly stroke, eliminate it from your workout until after the baby is born. Since the butterfly is very strenuous and requires an arched back, it is a poor choice for pregnant women. Some advanced swimmers may use the butterfly stroke into their pregnancies, but they will have to stop during their third trimesters. Your body will tell you when it's time to stop.

Although you're "eating for two" while you're pregnant you don't have to drastically increase the amount of food you eat. Consult your doctor. You may wish to increase your intake of fresh fruits, fluids, vegetables, and whole grains. If you're unaccustomed to exercise, you *may* have to increase the amount you eat to supply the extra calories you will burn off while in the water. But you should avoid junk food, processed food, food additives, caffeine, salt, tobacco, and alcohol. Don't swim immediately after eating a heavy meal.

As more women exercise throughout their childbearing years, the information available on pregnancy and fitness is increasing. Jane E. Brody, personal health writer for the *New York Times*, recently (February 2, 1994) emphasized that swimming and water exercise are ideal, if the water is neither very warm nor very cold, because the water supports your increasing weight and allows you to work out as vigorously in the ninth month as in the third. She stressed, however, that water skiing, scuba diving, and surfing are too risky at any stage of pregnancy and that diving and jumping should be avoided during the last trimester. She also stressed the importance of drinking enough water or caffeine-free liquid to avoid becoming overheated during exercise.

Other general safety tips to keep in mind include entering the pool by carefully climbing down the ladder or stairs or by sliding carefully into the pool from a sitting position on the wall. Do not jump, dive, or use any strenuous wall push-off because the impact of the water could cause stress to the uterus or to the fetus. You should never swim alone and never indulge in alcohol while swimming. You should leave the water if you feel chilly or numb or if your lips or fingers become blue.

General Workout Tips

The American College of Obstetricians and Gynecologists (ACOG) has developed guidelines for exercise safety during pregnancy and the postpartum period. Here is a summary of the ACOG recommendations that pertain to water fitness.

Pregnancy and Postpartum

1. Regular exercise (at least three times weekly) is preferable to intermittent activity.
2. Avoid vigorous exercise in hot, humid weather or when you are running a fever.
3. Avoid ballistic (jerky or bouncy) movements.
4. Avoid deep flexion or extension of joints because of connective tissue laxity. Avoid activities that require jumping, jarring motions, or rapid changes in direction because of joint instability.

5. Connective tissue laxity increases the risk of joint injury, so don't take stretches to the point of maximum resistance.
6. Precede vigorous exercise with a 5-minute warm-up period. Follow vigorous exercise with a period of gradually declining activity that includes gentle stationary stretching.
7. Measure heart rate at times of peak activity and avoid exceeding target heart rates and limits established in consultation with your physician.
8. Drink liquids liberally before and after exercise to prevent dehydration. If necessary, interrupt activity to replenish fluids.
9. If you have a sedentary lifestyle, begin with low-intensity physical activity and advance levels gradually.
10. Stop activity and consult your physician if any unusual symptoms appear.

Pregnancy Only

1. Limit maternal heart rate to not more than 140 beats per minute.
2. Limit strenuous activities to 15 minutes in duration.
3. Don't exercise in the supine position after the fourth month of gestation.
4. Avoid exercises that employ the Valsalva maneuver.
5. Make sure caloric intake is adequate to meet not only the extra energy needs of pregnancy, but also of the exercise performed.
6. Keep maternal core temperature at or below 38 °C.

These guidelines were originally published in 1985. Since then, new information about the responses of a pregnant woman and her baby to exercise has become available. Women who began pregnancy already fit and participating in vigorous activity felt that the original guidelines were too conservative. The new findings indicate the following:

1. Women who had been exercising previous to becoming pregnant were better able to respond to heat or cold.
2. Fetal breathing and body movements increased during exercise, indicating fetal well-being.
3. Babies born to women who exercised were within a normal range of birth weights.

The summary of a recent study in the *Physical Education Journal of Sports Medicine* (1993) indicated that pregnant women can exercise safely with minimal risk to themselves and their babies. Although they may not have been able to exercise at prepregnancy levels, they still derived benefits from being active. Exercise helped control hyperinsulinemia and weight gain, and the women felt better emotionally. Remember, however, to consult a physician before beginning a strenuous program.

Other general guidelines can help make your water fitness program beneficial and enjoyable.

- Exercise only as long as you remain comfortable; rest when you are tired and avoid straining.
- Perform each repetition of an exercise slowly and steadily. Concentrate on every movement and feel your body as it performs. Avoid pumping or jerky movements.
- Unless you are accustomed to vigorous exercise, start your program using five exercises, one from each of the exercise categories. Try to progress to spending 1 minute on each exercise.
- Breathe deeply, rhythmically, and continuously through each exercise; deep breathing enhances the pleasure and relaxation the exercises produce. (Be careful not to hyperventilate, however.)
- Begin and end each exercise with a cleansing breath to practice the cleansing breath for labor and delivery.
- Add effleurage (a light, gentle, fingertip massage) of the abdomen whenever possible, so that it will come naturally when you need it during labor and delivery.
- Exercise to music when possible, if you like.
- Avoid overstretching because your joints and ligaments are naturally relaxed during pregnancy. Avoid toe pointing, which can cause leg cramps.
- Wear a waterproof wristwatch to time your water exercise or use a clock in the pool area. A pace clock or a standard wall clock, preferably with a sweep second hand, is appropriate.
- Be creative—combine exercises and design a workout sequence and variations to fit your needs.
- Above all, relax, breathe deeply, and enjoy yourself during your water fitness workout.

Water Exercise Equipment

Now it's time to get ready to go into the pool. First, though, look over this list of things you'll need for either a water exercise workout or a swim workout (see Figure 2.1).

- A swimsuit. In your first trimester, your regular swimsuit will be adequate because your weight gain is usually minimal. In your second trimester, you may need a larger size or a swimsuit that will stretch. In your third trimester, use a leotard, a larger stretch suit, or a maternity suit. As your pregnancy progresses, your breasts will enlarge so you may want to wear a swimsuit with a soft-cup bra for comfort and support or perhaps a leotard with a bra underneath.

- Cap. If the pool regulations require a cap or if you choose to wear one, here are some pointers: If your hair is long, a cap of lycra rather than latex is easier to work with. If you want to keep your hair dry, wear a latex cap over the lycra cap. Silicone caps, which are smoother and cause less hair pulling, are also available.

Some swimmers apply a little baby oil or conditioner to their hair before swimming and wear a swim cap. Wash your hair after you swim. Because of the demands frequent swimming places on your hair, you may wish to choose a hairstyle that is manageable with frequent washings. Conditioners can be put on hair after swimming.

- A pair of goggles. Goggles are not absolutely necessary, especially if you are planning workouts exclusively of water exercise. Goggles do keep the pH of the water from bothering your eyes as you swim, and they improve vision in the water. (They'll open a whole new underwater world to you.) Goggles come in many different styles—the best way to choose the most comfortable style for you is simply to try on different types. Most goggles adjust at the nosepiece, the head strap, or both for comfort and a watertight fit. You can even buy goggles with prescription lenses if you need them. However, you'll find that ordinary goggles in the water have a refractive effect that ameliorates nearsightedness (and they're quite a bit less expensive).

- A waterproof wristwatch. Wear a waterproof watch with a sweep second hand or a digital watch with functions for seconds and a stopwatch. These will be a great help in timing your exercises.

Then there is some equipment you *might* like to try to add variety to your water exercises or swimming. Many facilities have this equipment available for their swimmers.

- A kickboard. This is a flat flotation device that you can use to support your body while kicking. It is also used in certain water exercises.

- A pull-buoy. This is a small flotation device that you can use to add resistance in many water exercises. Its primary purpose is to support your legs while you're practicing arm strokes.

- Swim fins. These large paddles, often used in skin diving and scuba diving, attach to your feet. In the pool, they are great for exercising your hips and legs because they greatly increase resistance. Swim fins work best with the flutter kick and will make you fly through the water. In case you've never tried them, they are *lots of fun*!

- Hand paddles. These hard plastic disks attach to your hands to increase resistance. They work to strengthen your arms and shoulders the way swim fins work for your hips and legs. You can also use mitts or gloves.

Starting Properly, Getting Equipped 19

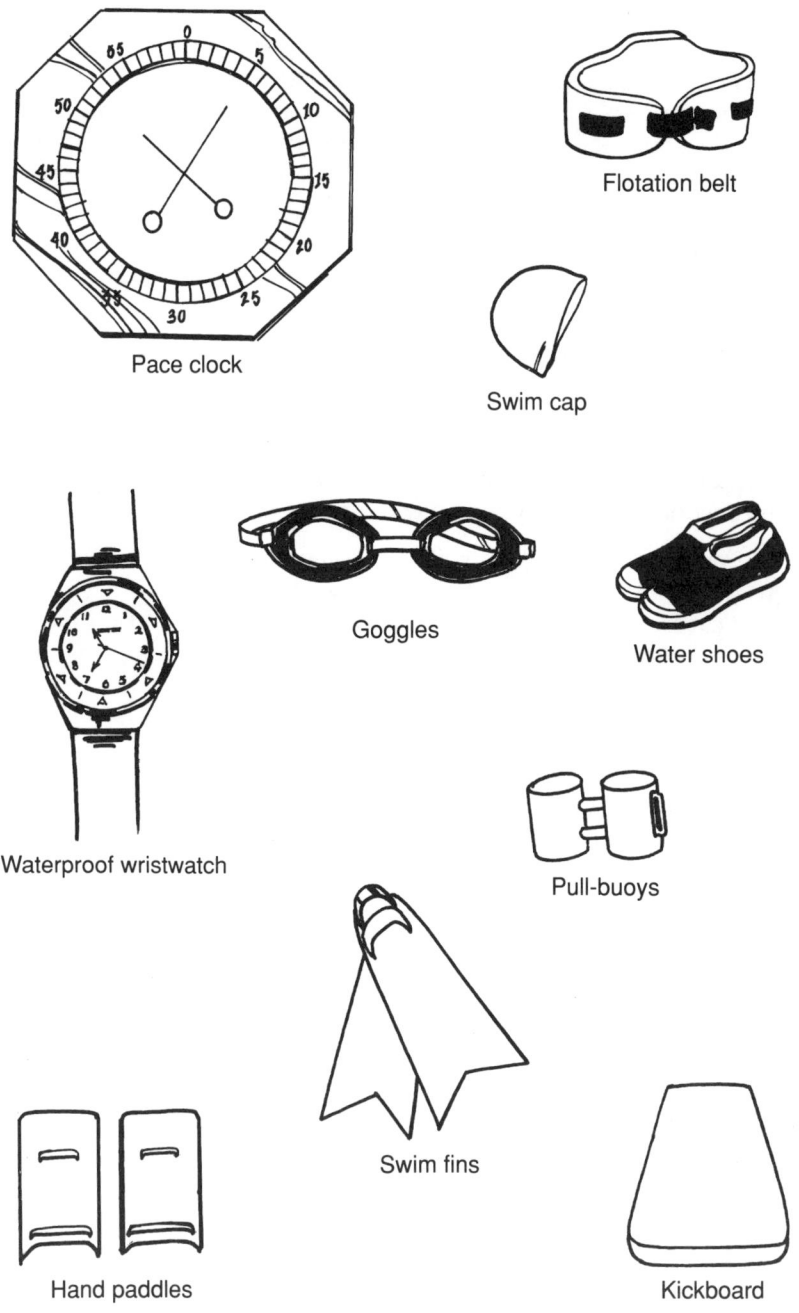

Figure 2.1 Water exercise equipment.

- Water shoes. These are shoes made of waterproof fabric (usually some form of rubber and/or nylon) with textured rubber soles to provide traction. Wearing water shoes is an important preventive measure to help you keep your balance. Water shoes also help prevent slipping in the locker area or pool deck. They can be worn in the pool during exercise to provide your feet with traction, cushioning and support, as well as protection from injuries from accidentally walking on sharp objects.
- Flotation supports. These flotation devices (e.g., belts or vests) are made of buoyant material. They support your body in the water, enabling you to exercise in an upright position. They are especially useful for deep-water exercise such as deep-water walking or jogging.
- A pace clock. Most swimming facilities are equipped with a large timing clock with a sweep second hand called a pace clock. This clock is ideal for timing your water exercises, swims, and rest periods. Learning to use the clock also prepares you to time your labor contractions. (If your facility doesn't have a pace clock, it may have a large wall clock with a sweep second hand that you can use for timing.)

This swim gear is readily available. Some sources for swimwear and swim equipment follow. This is not an exhaustive list, but it is a good start. In most cases, a catalog (some of them free) is available upon request.

Arena USA
6900 S. Peoria St.
Englewood, CO 80112
303-799-1856

Head Sports Wear
9189 Red Branch Rd.
Columbia, MD 21045
410-730-8300

Herman's "We Are Sports"
2 Germack Dr.
Carteret, NJ 07008
908-541-1550

Kast-a-Way Swimwear, Inc.
9356 Cincinnati/Columbus Rd.
Cincinnati, OH 45241
1-800-543-2763

Lady Madonna Maternity Boutiques
793 Madison Ave.
New York, NY 10021
212-988-7173

Maternity fashions (includes Reborn Maternity, Maternity Ltd., Maternity Warehouse, Expecting the Best)
1-800-USA-MOMS (800-872-6667)

Motherhood Maternity Boutiques
390 N. Sepulveda Blvd.
El Segundo, CA 90245

Speedo/Authentic Fitness
6040 Bandini Blvd.
Los Angeles, CA 90040
213-726-1262

Suits Me Swimwear
2377 Deltona Blvd.
Spring Hill, FL 34606
904-666-1485

World Wide Aquatics
10500 University Center Dr., Ste. 250
Tampa, FL 33612
1-800-726-1530

Also, check your local Yellow Pages for sporting goods and department stores, apparel shops, and boutiques for maternity sports wear, as well as your local Speedo/Authentic retailer.

Now that you know what guidelines to follow and what equipment to use in your water exercise program, you are ready to learn the exercises in Part II.

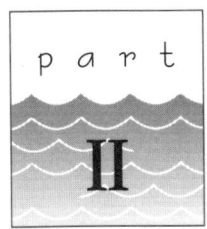

WATER EXERCISE TECHNIQUES: THE W.E.T. WORKOUT PROGRAM FOR PREGNANCY

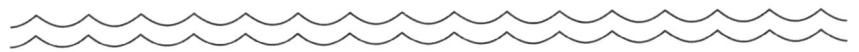

Water Exercise Techniques (WET) are a series of firming, strengthening, and stretching exercises performed in the water. Exercising with the W.E.T. Workout is comfortable because it can accommodate the increase in your body volume and buoyancy as your pregnancy progresses. WETs complement prepared childbirth programs by working different parts of the body to increase strength and flexibility, maintaining your conditioning level, and preparing you for labor and delivery. The exercises also give you practice in using the cleansing breath and effleurage, which are labor techniques, and teach you how to concentrate on your body's movements and how to relax.

Both swimmers and nonswimmers can enjoy the refreshing advantage of a water workout. Select exercises appropriate to your fitness level, your swimming skills, and the stage of your pregnancy. WETs are ideal for exercising in a pool that is too small for swimming laps, irregularly shaped, or too crowded for swimming laps. WETs are also appropriate when you are too tired to swim laps comfortably. On those days, you can adjust the number of repetitions or duration of each exercise to your comfort level. This is helpful if your energy or motivation to swim is low, but you want to conscientiously maintain your conditioning.

During your postpartum period, return to the water with WETs, either as the main set of your workout or for the warm-up and stretch-out segments of your lap swimming workout.

Part II contains six chapters of water exercises. To start with, you'll find warm-up and cool-down exercises in chapter 3 and breathing exercises in chapter 4. These chapters are followed by upper-, middle-, lower-, and total-body exercises, which will be used in the main set of your workouts. You can mix and match individual exercises to create your own WET workout, or you can follow the sample workouts in Part IV. Use common sense in your choices and you will find that water exercises are fun and relaxing as well as very beneficial.

chapter 3

WARM-UP AND COOL-DOWN EXERCISES

The right way—very likely, that's how your mother taught you to do things. Now more than ever you are concerned about doing things the safe way. Although the preferred way of doing any activity actually can be subject to differences of opinion, exercising in preparation for childbirth is one activity that must be done *the right way.*

The right way to work out—whether you are pregnant or not—is to include three basic elements of workouts in *every* workout session. Every workout, on land or in water, should include these components: a warm-up, the main set, and a cool-down followed by stretching. These components ensure both optimum performance—making the best use of your workout time and effort—and physical safety. It is all the more important to follow this pattern while you are pregnant.

The *warm-up* is a 5- to 10-minute session that prepares your muscles and cardiorespiratory system for working out by slowly loosening and stretching your muscles, slightly elevating your heart rate, and easing your joints into an exercise mode. Although your actual physical exertion during this period is relatively light, the warm-up enables you to adjust mentally and physically from a "resting" condition in a land environment to a water workout. You might think that this time is not well spent, but it is. *Don't skip your warm-up!*

The *main set* is the aerobic part of the workout, which usually consists of about 20 minutes of active movement in the water designed to exercise all areas of your body. Generally, you exert the most concentrated effort during the main set, elevating your heart rate. Elevating your heart rate is not the goal of exercising during pregnancy as it is at other times, but your heart rate will still increase slightly during the main set.

Try to vary the exercises in your main set so that you regularly perform exercises from each of the five categories of water exercises: breathing exercises, upper-body exercises, middle-body exercises, lower-body exercises, and total-body exercises.

The *cool-down* concludes the workout with approximately 5 minutes of easy stretches and posture exercises to gradually return the body to its warm-up state and heart rate.

Exercise physiologists recommend that exercises that move (and warm up) your muscles *precede* stretching exercises. With that in mind, use the following 10 exercises at the beginning and end of each workout according to your fitness level, stage of pregnancy, and personal preference.

Warm-Up, Cool-Down Exercises 27

1

OVERHEAD STRETCH

Benefits

Begins stretching the muscles in preparation for the workout.

Equipment

One towel

Starting Position

Stand on the pool deck with feet hip-width apart before going into the pool for this dry-land stretch.

How to Do It

1. Roll up your towel, grasp an end in each hand, and place it behind your neck. Extend your arms with the towel taut between them over your head, and stretch your body by moving gradually from left to right, keeping your arms straight. Breathe normally; do not hold your breath.

2. Then, without your towel, extend your left arm over your head, palm facing in. Again, breathe normally.

3. Bend your left elbow and grasp it from the front with your right hand. Guide the left arm to reach behind your head, resting your hand at the base of your neck. Gently pull on your left elbow for additional stretch.

4. Release and reverse arms.

2

SIT AND KICK

Benefits

Helps you get used to the water, and prepares the legs for the workout. This also makes weary feet feel great.

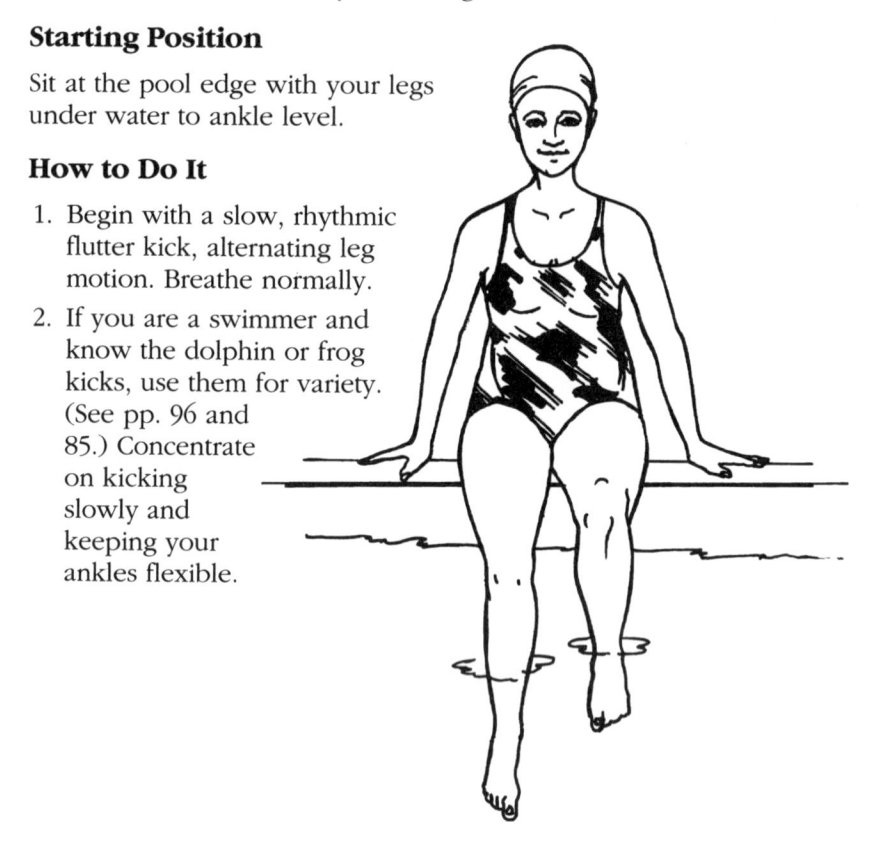

Starting Position

Sit at the pool edge with your legs under water to ankle level.

How to Do It

1. Begin with a slow, rhythmic flutter kick, alternating leg motion. Breathe normally.
2. If you are a swimmer and know the dolphin or frog kicks, use them for variety. (See pp. 96 and 85.) Concentrate on kicking slowly and keeping your ankles flexible.

FEET FLEX

Benefits

Stretches your calf muscles.

Starting Position

Sit at the edge of the pool with your legs extended forward in the water.

How to Do It

1. Gently flex your feet toward the ceiling, then point your toes forward. Breathe normally.
2. Repeat.

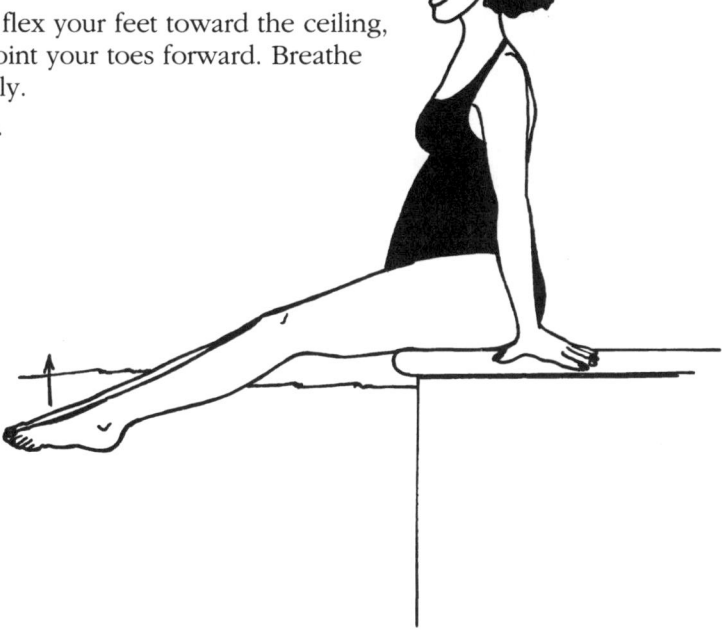

4

WATER WALK/JOG

Benefits

Helps your body adjust to the water, water temperature, and water resistance.

Starting Position

Stand in chest-deep water, knees slightly bent.

How to Do It

1. Walk through the water, moving your arms back and forth. Breathe normally.
2. You can travel forward, backward, diagonally, or in a circle, and you can try varying the size of your steps. If you feel energetic, switch into an easy jog, then return to walking.

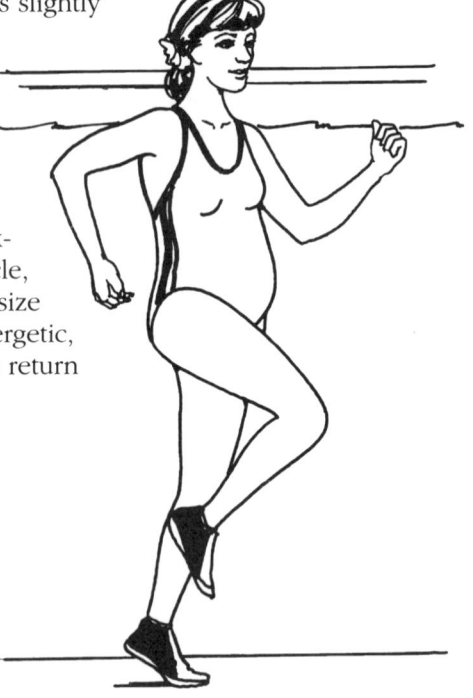

SHOULDER SHRUG

Benefits

Loosens and relieves tension in your shoulders.

Starting Position

Stand in chest-deep water with arms relaxed at your sides, knees slightly bent, and legs hip-width apart.

How to Do It

1. Lift both shoulders up toward your ears.
2. Roll them alternately forward several times, then back several times. Then roll both shoulders together. Breathe normally.

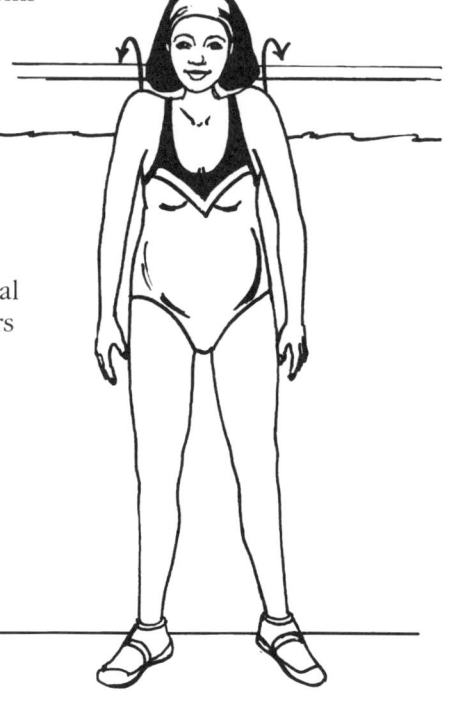

6

STAND TALL

Benefits

Helps in body alignment, which is a major factor in comfort during your pregnancy (see p. 55), and relieves strain on back muscles.

Starting Position

Stand in chest-deep water with your shoulders, back, buttocks, and heels against the pool wall. Place feet as close together as possible, and keep your arms at your side.

How to Do It

1. Take one step away from the wall, keeping your posture the same. Do not hold your breath—breathe normally.
2. Return to the wall and recheck your position.

7

PELVIC TILT

Benefits

Helps in body alignment, relieves strain on back muscles, and strengthens abdominal muscles.

Starting Position

Stand in waist-deep water with your back and hips against the pool wall. Place your feet as close together as possible. Rest your arms on the pool ledge for support.

How to Do It

1. Tilt your pelvis upward by pressing the small of your back toward the wall.
2. Face down. Hold for a moment, then slowly relax back to the starting position. Breathe normally.

WATER KEGEL

Benefits

Isolates and strengthens the perineal and pelvic floor muscles, giving better support of your reproductive organs, and improving your control during delivery. The Kegel exercise develops improved circulation in the perineum, aiding the healing process after birth and helping to relieve discomfort of hemorrhoids during your recovery. If done regularly, the Kegel exercise can help prevent urinary incontinence both during and after your pregnancy. Kegels should be included in every workout.

Equipment

Flotation support (optional)

Starting Position

Stand in chest-deep water with your feet less than hip-width apart.

How to Do It

1. Tighten your lower abdominal muscles, then contract your pelvic floor and vaginal muscles. Release your muscles. After 10 repetitions, hold the contraction and your breath for 5 to 10 seconds, then release and exhale.
2. You can repeat the sequence several times during your workout.
3. You can also use a flotation support to allow your feet to float off the pool bottom.

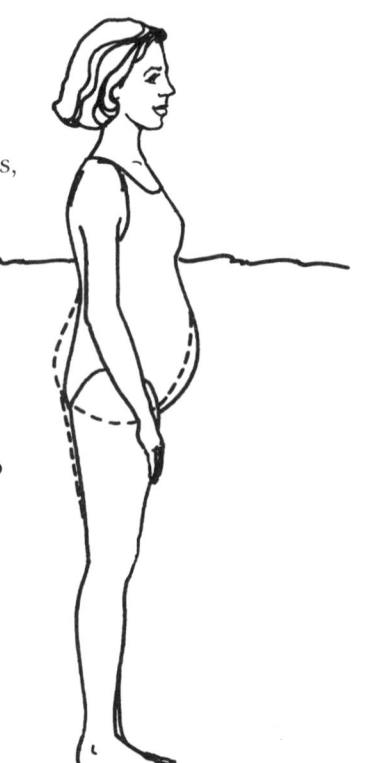

Warm-Up, Cool-Down Exercises 35

9

AQUA LUNGE

Benefits

Stretches your inner- and outer-thigh muscles.

Starting Position

Face the pool wall and hold the edge with both hands shoulder-width apart. Place your feet more than shoulder-width apart against the wall in a straddle position.

How to Do It

1. Shift your weight to the right side, bending the right knee, and extend the left leg. Hold for 10-20 seconds.
2. Return to the center and shift your weight to the other side. Breathe normally.

Exercise Tip

- Your hip joints are relaxed during pregnancy, so be careful not to overstretch.

10

EFFLEURAGE

Benefits

Helps you relax during labor and delivery by diverting your mind somewhat from the pain of the internal contraction. This prepared childbirth technique is usually combined with a breathing exercise.

Starting Position

Stand in the pool at any comfortable water depth or float on your back.

How to Do It

1. Place your fingers on your navel, pointed slightly downward.
2. Trace a circular design on your abdomen with your fingertips in a continuous motion for approximately one minute.

Exercise Tip

- In the Lamaze method, effleurage becomes a conditioned reaction to any tightness in the abdomen as pregnancy progresses. You can also use effleurage between exercises and with different breathing patterns.

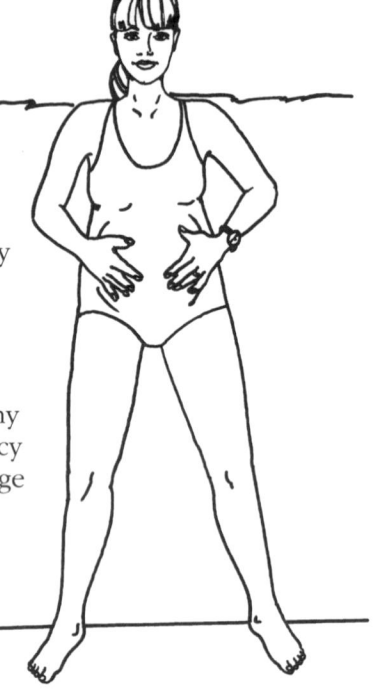

chapter 4

BREATHING EXERCISES

Breathing is basic. Controlled breathing is a key element of prepared childbirth. Following are Water Exercise Techniques you should incorporate into your water fitness workout to help you control your breathing.

These five exercises correspond to Lamaze breathing, so they can help develop your breathing technique for childbirth and help you achieve a more complete air exchange. Your ability to breathe deeply and fully, with an expanded lung capacity, may help you manage pain during labor and delivery.

Include the breathing exercises as part of your workout warm-up, in addition to the exercises in chapter 3. As a reminder, during your warm-up, do the *warming-up* exercises before the *stretching* exercises.

11

CLEANSING BREATH

Benefits

Develops your ability to breathe deeply and fully. The cleansing breath is used during labor at the beginning and end of each contraction.

Starting Position

Stand in the pool in waist- to chest-deep water with your arms extended out to the sides, legs comfortably spaced.

How to Do It

1. Inhale deeply and slowly through your nose, then exhale slowly and completely through your mouth.
2. Do five repetitions, rest, and repeat.

Exercise Tip

- The cleansing breath can be done before and after every warm-up period and cool-down period of your workout.

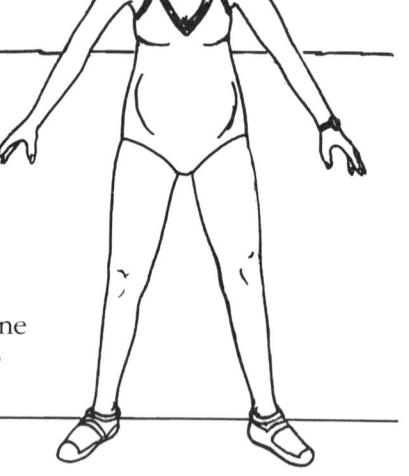

Variation

- Stand in chest-deep water, holding on to the pool wall with one hand and bending your knees so that your face is just above the surface. Inhale through your nose, then put your face into the water and exhale simultaneously through your nose and mouth.

12

BREATHE AND REACH

Benefits

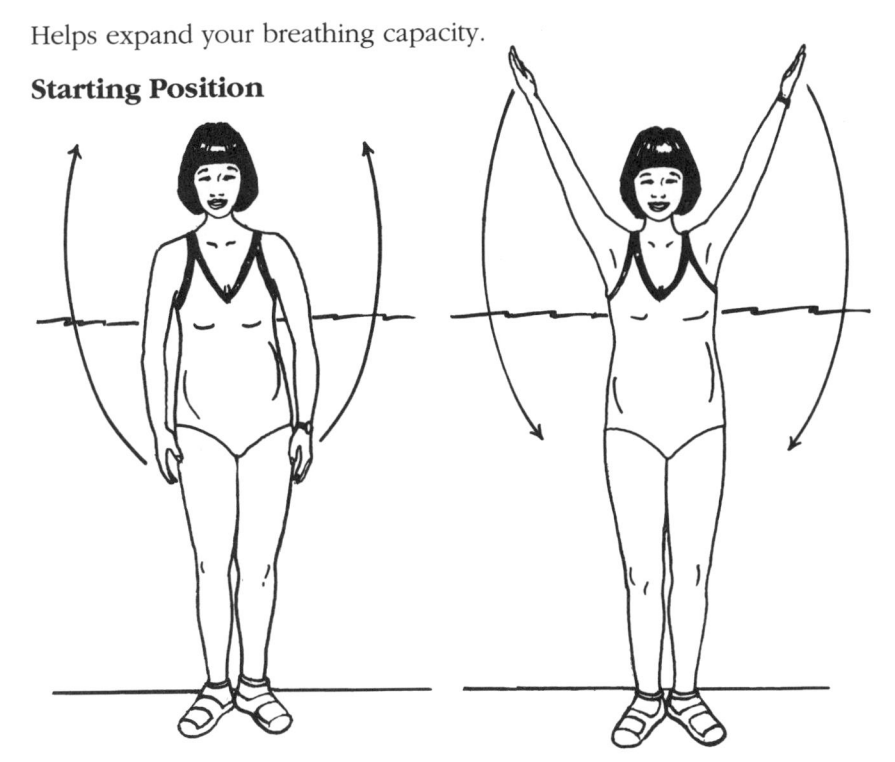

Helps expand your breathing capacity.

Starting Position

Stand in waist-deep water with your arms at your sides and feet together.

How to Do It

1. Lift your arms to an overhead position to inhale, turning your palms up.
2. With your arms extended overhead, alternately stretch them upward a few times.
3. Then slowly return your arms to the starting position as you exhale.

Exercise Tip

- During the early stages of your pregnancy, cross your arms in front of you as you inhale and raise your arms overhead as you exhale.

Breathing With Head Circles

Benefits

Helps tone and stretch your head and neck muscles and helps relieve muscle tension in the head and neck areas.

Starting Position

Stand in neck-deep water, feet hip-width apart, with your head facing forward. Place your hands at your sides or rest them lightly on your hips.

How to Do It

1. Slowly rotate your head in one direction, inhaling deeply through your nose and mouth, until you have turned your head in a quarter circle.
2. Then exhale through your nose and mouth as you turn your head back to its original position.
3. Repeat the exercise, moving your head in the other direction.

Exercise Tip

- Add your cleansing breath to your head circles by inhaling through your nose and exhaling through your mouth.
- Avoid hyperextending your head and neck backward. Keep the movement to a quarter circle.

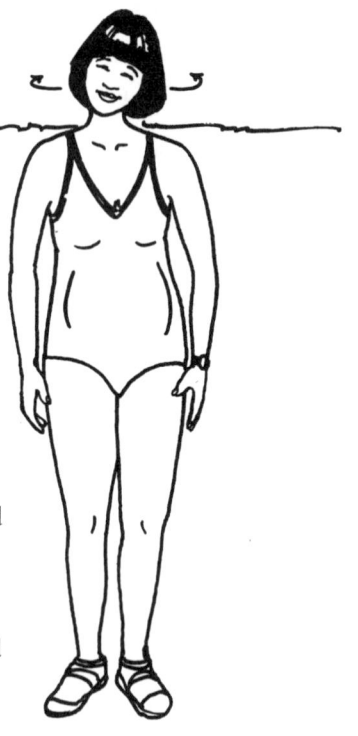

14

BREATHE AND BOB

Benefits
Develops general breathing technique and increases breath control.

Starting Position
Stand in chest-deep water with one leg slightly in front of the other, hip-width apart. Keep arms underwater for balance.

How to Do It

1. Inhale deeply through your nose and mouth, then exhale slowly and completely through your nose and mouth.
2. Combine your breathing with bobbing. Inhale just before bending your knees to submerge. Exhale continuously through your nose and mouth underwater. Then, still exhaling, straighten your knees to emerge from the water. Repeat.

Exercise Tips

- Practice controlled breathing by deliberately timing your exhalations so they take more time than your inhalations.
- Hold onto the pool wall or ladder for support while you're standing or bobbing.
- You can supplement your breathing exercises by doing crawl and breaststroke arm motions while breathing.

15

LABOR AND DELIVERY BREATHING PATTERNS

Benefits

Develops the Lamaze breathing techniques you will use during labor and delivery and increases breath control.

Starting Position

Stand in chest-deep water, legs comfortably spaced and knees slightly bent.

How to Do It

1. To practice the *cleansing breath* used during labor and at the beginning and end of each contraction (see p. 38), inhale deeply and slowly through your nose, then exhale slowly and completely through your mouth. Breathe twice at the beginning and end of each of the other breathing exercises.
2. To practice for breathing during the *early stages of labor*, breathe using *slow chest breathing* (deep, full chest expansion) at a rate of six to nine breaths per minute. Repeat for 1 minute.
3. To practice for *breathing during transition*, combine panting breaths (short, shallow breaths) with a deep, full exhalation (a "blow"); do four to six pants, then a blow. Repeat for 1-1/2 minutes.
4. To practice for *pushing* and birth, use a sequence of two quick cleansing breaths, followed by a deep inhalation through the nose that you hold 5 to 10 seconds before a deep exhalation through the mouth. Repeat for 1-1/2 minutes.

Exercise Tips

- Remember to begin and end each breathing exercise with a cleansing breath.
- Use the accompanying chart (Table 4.1) to remind you of the Lamaze breathing patterns you will use during labor and delivery.
- Practice the breathing pattern for the early stages of labor while you are doing your water exercises or lap swimming.
- Practice transition breathing while doing the breaststroke or sidestroke.

Table 4.1 Breathing Patterns Used During Labor and Delivery

Stage of labor	Approximate time	Frequency of contractions	Duration of contractions	Intensity of contractions	Dilation	Type of breathing used
1st—Early	8-10 hours	20 min	30-45 sec	Mild to moderate	0-4 cm	6-9 breaths per minute (slow chest)
Active	4-5 hours	2-3 min	45 sec-1 min	Moderate to intense	4-8 cm	Rapid/shallow chest (pants—he-he)
Transition	½ hour-1 hour	1-1½ min	1-2 min	Intense	8-10 cm	Rapid chest and blow (4-6 pants and blow)
2nd—Pushing to Birth	2 minutes to 3 hours	2-3 min	1-1½ min	Intense	10 cm	2 quick cleansing breaths; on 3rd, hold and push—breathe in and repeat (deep inhalation, approximately 5-10 seconds of holding; push down and out—release and repeat)
3rd—Afterbirth	5-30 min	2-3 min	1-1½ min	Mild to moderate	10 cm	Same as the pushing techniques and relaxation techniques

Note. From *Swimming Through Your Pregnancy* (p. 62) by J. Katz, 1983, New York: Doubleday. Copyright 1983 by Jane Katz. Reprinted by permission.

chapter 5

UPPER-BODY EXERCISES

Upper-body Water Exercise Techniques help stretch and strengthen your shoulders, arms, neck, chest, and upper back for one of the most demanding days of your life—the birth of your baby—and what may be one of your most challenging jobs—caring for your newborn baby.

Upper-body stretching exercises help you identify and reduce upper-body tension. Strengthened chest muscles (pectorals) also will help support your breasts as they increase in size, a factor in returning to your prepregnancy figure. Because overall toning during pregnancy helps provide the comfort and health advantages of maintaining good posture, the upper body is the place to begin.

Upper-body strength (trapezius, latissimus dorsi, and sternocleidomastoid muscles) will be important if you rely on your arms for support while in labor, or pushing during delivery (the need for this will depend on the facilities of your labor or birthing room).

Strong arms (biceps and triceps muscles) and shoulders (deltoid muscles) are especially important after birth because the abdominal muscles will be somewhat relaxed from the pregnancy, and they will not provide as much support as they would ordinarily. You'll need strength in your arms and shoulders to lift, hold, and carry your baby after the birth, as well as to lift, hold, and carry the baby's gear—baby bag, car seat, and bassinet, just for starters. As your baby grows you may also tote a stroller, walker, portable crib, and similar equipment. After that come scooter toys, three-wheelers, and the like. The practical aspects of motherhood consist of a myriad of tasks. Strengthening your upper body with the eight exercises in this chapter will help you to handle them without unnecessary discomfort and fatigue. So here are exercises to prepare you for pregnancy and parenthood. (Perhaps your partner or coach should join you in them!)

16

MEDLEY OF PULLS

Benefits

Tones and strengthens all your upper-body muscles while reviewing the major swim strokes.

Starting Position

Stand in chest-deep water with feet spaced comfortably apart.

How to Do It

Do 10 arm stroke cycles for each of the following:

1. Crawl stroke—hand-over-hand alternating forward circular motion, with an overarm recovery. Coordinate breathing with your arm motion.
2. Breaststroke—rhythmic heart-shaped pull simultaneously with both arms, with underwater recovery. Inhale as you pull and exhale as you recover.
3. Sidestroke—bring hands together at chest, palms together, and then separate your arms, moving one arm overhead and the other to your side. Inhale as hands come together and exhale as they extend.
4. Backstroke—alternating back windmill motion. Breathe normally.

Exercise Tips

- Balance your body by placing one foot in front of the other.
- Alternate stroke speeds (e.g., do five easy strokes followed by five vigorous strokes).
- Create your own sequence of arm strokes.

17

ARM PRESS

Benefits

Tones and strengthens upper-body muscles, promotes upper-body flexibility, and helps you identify and control upper-body tension.

Equipment

Hand paddles (optional)

Starting Position

Stand in chin-deep water, feet as close together as possible. Extend your right arm in front of you at shoulder height with your palm facing down. Extend your left arm behind you at shoulder height with your palm facing down.

How to Do It

1. Press both of your hands down toward your thighs and then upward in an arc so that you finish with the right arm extended behind you and your left arm extended in front of you.
2. Turn your palms so they face down (again) and repeat.
3. Add your cleansing breath. Breathe in through your nose and out through your mouth on succeeding arm presses.

Exercise Tips

- Keep your feet spread apart and your knees slightly bent to help you maintain your balance. To increase the difficulty of the exercise, use hand paddles.
- Perform these exercises slowly.

Variation

- Extend both arms in front of you at shoulder height with your palms facing outward. Press your arms away from each other (strengthening your triceps muscles and forearms) until they are extended out to your sides.
- Then turn your hands over and press your arms together until your palms meet.
- Add your cleansing breath. Breathe in through your nose and out through your mouth on succeeding arm presses.
- For variety, combine one or both exercises with knee bends.

18

ARM CIRCLE

Benefits
Develops your shoulder, arm, and upper-back strength.

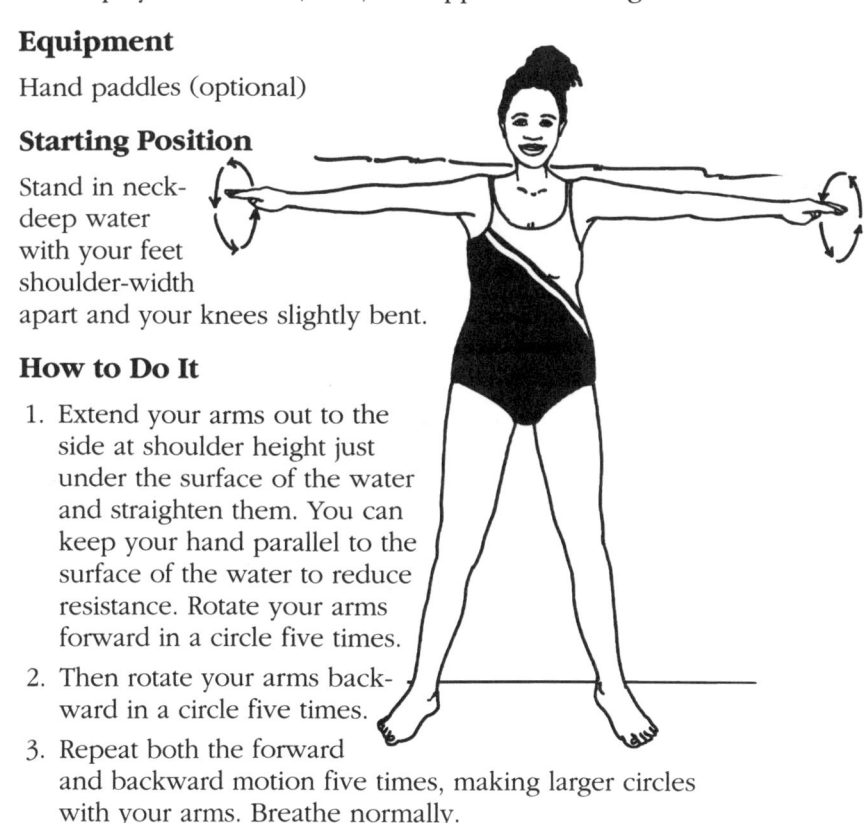

Equipment
Hand paddles (optional)

Starting Position
Stand in neck-deep water with your feet shoulder-width apart and your knees slightly bent.

How to Do It
1. Extend your arms out to the side at shoulder height just under the surface of the water and straighten them. You can keep your hand parallel to the surface of the water to reduce resistance. Rotate your arms forward in a circle five times.
2. Then rotate your arms backward in a circle five times.
3. Repeat both the forward and backward motion five times, making larger circles with your arms. Breathe normally.

Exercise Tips
- For added resistance, use hand paddles while doing the exercise with small circles.
- Use arm circles as a warm-up exercise for the crawl stroke. Avoid ballistic movements.

Variation
- Place your hands on your shoulders and rotate your arms at the shoulder, moving your arms in a circle (like chicken wings).

SPORT SWING

Benefits
Tones and strengthens the upper body muscles.

Equipment
Hand paddles (optional)

Starting Position
Stand in chest-deep water with knees and hips slightly flexed, legs hip-width apart.

How to Do It
1. Extend your arms in front of you at shoulder height and clasp your palms underwater.
2. Turn your torso to the right, keeping your feet motionless and pulling on your left hand with your right hand.
3. Then turn to the left, pulling on your right hand with your left hand.
4. Remember to breathe deeply and continuously.

Exercise Tips
- Hand paddles increase resistance as you bring your arms through the water.
- Allowing the heel of your "trailing" leg to lift and turn will allow full range of motion.

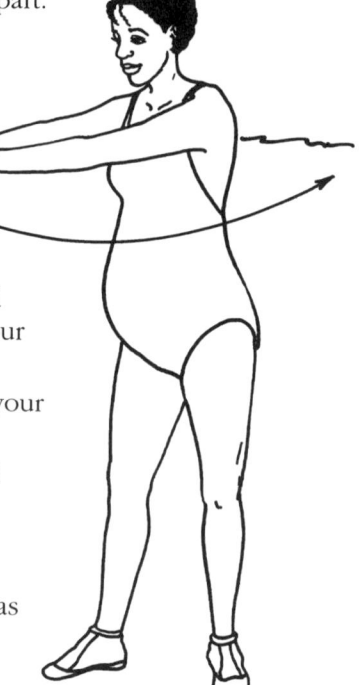

HANG 10

Benefits

Stretches and relaxes the upper body, helping to relax your neck.

Starting Position

Stand with your back against the pool wall.

How to Do It

1. Reach over your shoulders and grasp the pool edge with your hands more than shoulder-width apart.
2. Bend your knees so that your feet lift off the pool bottom, allowing the weight of your body to stretch your arms and upper body.
3. Relax your head and neck muscles and breathe deeply as you stretch. Hold stretch for 5 to 10 seconds.

Exercise Tips

- Use extra caution to avoid overstretching the tissue around the shoulder area—remember that your joints relax during pregnancy.
- To increase the stretch, move your hands closer together.
- Use the corner of the pool for greater comfort and support.

21

SCULLING

Benefits

Helps to ease neck tension and gently tones the upper-body muscles, especially those of the chest that help support your breasts. Sculling is a basic skill used in synchronized swimming.

Equipment

Hand paddles (optional)

Starting Position

Stand in shoulder-deep water with your feet almost together, knees bent. Extend your arms behind your hips under the surface and close to each other.

How to Do It

1. Move your hands in a figure-eight motion: turn your palms downward and outward and press your hands out past shoulder width, keeping your upper arms relatively motionless.
2. Then turn your palms inward and press your hands in until they almost touch.
3. Then turn your palms outward and repeat the movement.
4. Breathe slowly in and out through your nose and mouth as you scull.

Variation

- Stand in shoulder-deep water, knees bent, with your arms extended forward under the surface of the water. Practice figure-eight sculling arm motion. Paddles are optional.

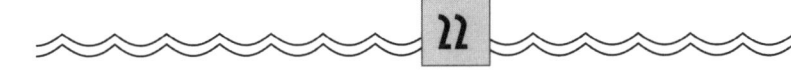

WALL PUSH-UP

Benefits

Strengthens the shoulders, arms, and chest muscles.

Starting Position

Stand in chest-deep water facing the pool wall. Your feet should be far enough away from the wall so that you can just reach the edge of the pool. Grasp the pool edge with your hands shoulder-width apart.

How to Do It

1. Slowly bend your elbows, keeping your body straight and your feet stationary until your chin approaches the pool edge.
2. Then slowly straighten your arms until you resume a standing position.
3. Inhale through your nose as you bend your elbows, and exhale through your mouth as you straighten your arms.

Exercise Tip

- Bend and straighten your arms slowly to increase the duration of the exercise. Moving slowly is also safer because you can more easily control your body.

KICKBOARD PRESS

Benefits
Strengthens shoulder, arm, and chest muscles by working against the resistance of the water on the kickboard.

Equipment
Kickboard

Starting Position
Stand in chest-deep water with your hands on a kickboard held widthwise.

How to Do It
1. Slowly straighten your arms and push the board under the water. Follow your normal breathing pattern.
2. Slowly allow the board to return to the surface.

Variation
- During your third trimester, you can vary this exercise by holding the board widthwise over your head. Lower it slowly, with arms extended, to touch the surface of the water. Return to overhead stretched position.

chapter 6

MIDDLE-BODY EXERCISES

These middle-body exercises will help you progress comfortably through pregnancy and will strengthen you for labor and delivery. Common complaints of pregnancy are lower-back discomfort and fatigue from carrying a growing abdomen. Middle-body exercises help strengthen the back (spinus erectus) and abdominal (oblique and transverse) muscles to support added weight and maintain good posture. Keeping your body aligned so your joints and muscles are not subject to unnecessary strain will help eliminate lower-back pain.

As your pregnancy progresses, your center of gravity—the theoretical center of body weight—moves forward. A strong back is essential for good posture during pregnancy because this shift in weight forces it to compensate for the stress. Any problem in body alignment is likely to cause back pain as your pregnancy progresses.

In addition, stretching and possible separation of your abdominal muscles and natural softening of ligaments caused by pregnancy hormones result in less support for your growing belly; not surprisingly, the abdominal muscles are those most stressed by pregnancy.

You can avoid much discomfort by strengthening abdominal muscles through exercise so back muscles need not be responsible for so much support. Toned muscles can carry more of the load; stretched muscles help you relax. Working these muscles helps maintain their elasticity, making them better able to support the pelvis and to return to normal after delivery.

Stretched and strengthened muscles are helpful in labor and delivery because you are more flexible and can better assist with pushing the baby from your body. After birth your exercise program will pay off again—you'll find it easier to get back into prepregnancy clothes, and your strong back and abdomen will be better equipped to lift the baby and gear.

24

CIRCLE SPRAY

Benefits
Tones the waist and torso while developing middle-body flexibility.

Starting Position
Stand in waist-deep water with your arms extended to your sides and your fingers at the water's surface. Stand with feet shoulder-width apart for balance, knees and hips slightly flexed.

How to Do It
1. Turn slowly in one direction as far as you can, keeping your feet stationary and your arms straight. Your fingertips should spray the water as you move. Breathe normally.
2. Twist your torso slowly back until you are facing front, then turn as far as you can in the opposite direction.
3. Slowly return again to the center position. Letting the heel of your trailing leg lift and turn will allow full range of motion.

Variation
- You can do this exercise while keeping your hands on your hips under the water.

HIP TOUCH

Benefits

Stretches and tones the abdominal muscles.

Starting Position

Stand in waist-deep water at almost arm's distance from the pool wall. Keep feet together. Grasp the pool edge with your inside hand, resting your lower arm on the edge.

How to Do It

1. Keeping your feet on the bottom, try to touch your hip to the wall, keeping your outside arm at water level.
2. Swing your hips as far away from the wall as possible. Breathe normally.
3. Repeat on the other side.

Variation

- For a greater stretch, when you swing your hips away from the wall, reach your outside arm overhead, toward the wall.

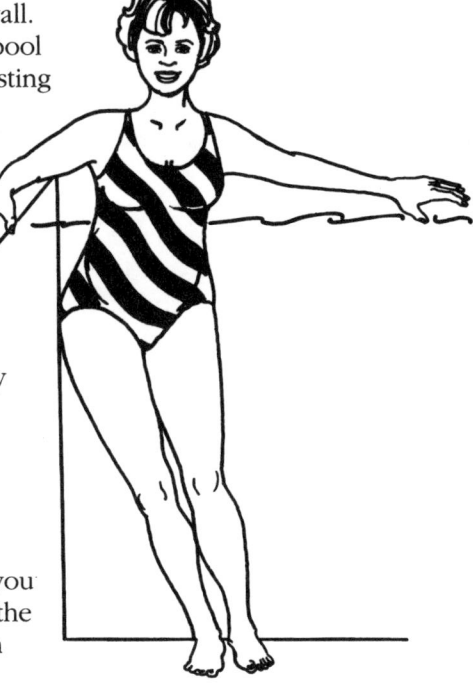

26

BACK EXTENSION

Benefits

Stretches the spine; relaxes the lower back and relieves pressure and discomfort there; strengthens the abdominal, back, and upper-thigh muscles; and helps develop concentration and body control.

Starting Position

Hold onto the pool wall with arms shoulder-width apart; place feet on the wall slightly farther apart than arms. (Try to place the entire sole of each foot on the wall.)

How to Do It

1. Slowly let your legs extend behind you into a prone float position. Inhale. Use your abdominal muscles to tilt your pelvis and control your legs until your feet are at the water's surface and separated slightly.
2. Stretch out and curl your back slowly (like a hissing cat). Feel the stretch completely through your spine while you bend your knees toward your chest. Exhale. Using your abdominal muscles to bring your feet to the wall, return to your starting position.

Exercise Tips

- Do not hyperextend your back. If you have had back problems in the past, ask your doctor's advice before doing this exercise.
- If the water level is well below the deck or pool edge, move your hands to a bracket position for better support. (Grasp the pool edge with one hand and place the other hand flat against the pool wall with fingertips pointed down.)

Variations

- For a more energetic exercise, place one foot in a flotation device to increase the effort needed to bring your feet to the wall, helping to strengthen your abdominal muscles. Control your legs as they return to the water's surface, being careful not to arch your back.
- End the last repetition of this exercise in the extended position. This will relieve stress on your back muscles.

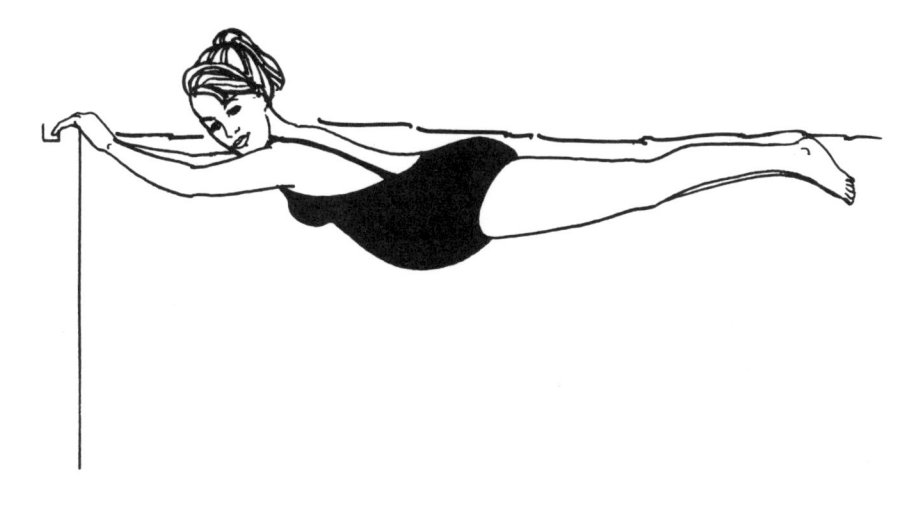

MODIFIED SIT-UP

Benefits

Strengthens and tones the muscles of the abdomen, hip flexors, and thighs.

Starting Position

Float on your back in chest-deep water with your neck resting on the pool edge. With arms extended to the sides, grasp the pool edge with both hands. Do the exercise in the corner of the pool if you need support.

How to Do It

1. Pull your knees to your chest.
2. Straighten your legs.
3. Breathe in through your nose as you draw your knees in, and out through your mouth as you straighten your legs.

Exercise Tips

- You can use this exercise throughout your pregnancy and during your postpartum period, with your doctor's approval. For maximum concentration on your abdominal muscles, be sure not to sit up too far.
- Modify starting position to comfortably adapt to water level and pool edge.

Variation

- Standing abdominal crunches can be done safely and comfortably during the early stages of pregnancy. As your pregnancy advances, you may be more comfortable bringing your knees over to one side.

28

SWING AND SWAY

Benefits
Stretches the torso, hips, and legs.

Starting Position
Face the pool wall and hold the edge with both hands shoulder-width apart and arms extended. Place your feet together on the pool floor.

How to Do It

1. Bending at the waist, walk up the wall with knees bent and apart until your feet are at hip level.

2. Then extend your knees, bringing your body away from the wall for a count of five. Flex your knees a few times, bringing your body slowly near and away from the wall. Breathe regularly.

3. Then swing your hips from side to side, feeling the stretch in your buttocks and upper legs.

Exercise Tips

- Be careful not to overstretch.
- As your pregnancy progresses, you may be comfortable omitting the second phase of flexing your knees. Go right into swinging your hips.
- It is more important to keep your feet on the wall than it is to keep your legs straight. Keep your knees bent—do not fully extend them.

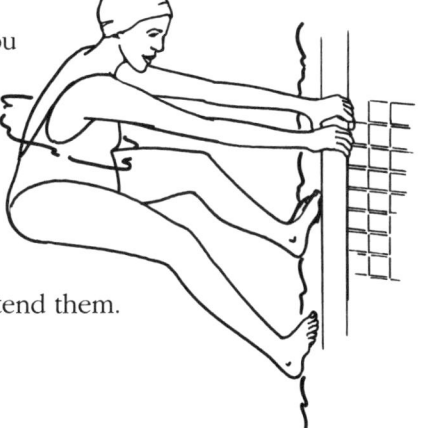

29

WALL KNEE LIFT

Benefits

Strengthens abdominal and back muscles, increases hip flexibility, and relaxes lower-back muscles.

Starting Position

Stand in chest-deep water with feet together and back against the pool wall. Hold onto the edge with your arms outstretched.

How to Do It

1. Tilt your pelvis forward and then back several times.
2. Then lift one knee up to waist level. Swing your knee toward the opposite shoulder, back to the front, out to the side away from the midline of your body, then back to center again. Slowly return the knee to starting position. Repeat on the other side.
3. Breathe slowly and regularly with each repetition.

Exercise Tips

- Keep your back and hips against the wall throughout this exercise.
- While turning your knees, do not lift your hips in the direction of the turn.

BACK MASSAGE

Benefits
Relaxes the back muscles.

Starting Position
Stand in shoulder-deep water, feet comfortably spaced, with your childbirth coach standing behind you.

How to Do It

1. Have your partner gently massage your back beneath the surface of the water.

2. Have your partner use the heels of the palms. Relax and breathe regularly. The back massage combined with the soothing properties of the water will make you feel wonderful!

Exercise Tips

- Try the Shoulder Shrug in conjunction with the massage. With your arms relaxed at your sides, roll your shoulders backward, then forward several times. Then lift and roll each shoulder separately. (See p. 31.)

- You can also use the Shoulder Shrug instead of the Back Massage if you are exercising without a partner.

chapter 7

LOWER-BODY EXERCISES

Lower-body exercises concentrate on hips, buttocks, and legs, helping make you more comfortable during pregnancy. Stretching and toning leg muscles in the water strengthens them to carry your increased load and helps alleviate pressure on the feet and ankles. Also, exercising in water helps eliminate excess fluid from the feet and ankles, reducing the discomfort of edema, which is common in mothers-to-be. In addition, exercising encourages increased circulation and discourages varicose veins.

Lower-body exercises mostly work your leg muscles (quadriceps and hamstrings for front and back thighs, abductor and adductor muscles for outer and inner thighs, and gastrocnemius muscles for your calves). Your lower abdominal muscles (transverse, oblique, and longitudinal muscles) also get a workout. As with middle-body exercises, strengthened abdominal muscles help you maintain good posture—a must for staying comfortable during pregnancy. Stronger abdominal muscles also provide assistance to the uterus during delivery.

This set of exercises includes specific techniques to stretch the pelvic floor muscles and inner thighs in preparation for delivery. While in labor, you may be asked to raise and open your legs in preparation for delivering your baby. By the time a vaginal birth is over, you will have stretched your inner thigh muscles for several hours. If you have been exercising your legs during your pregnancy, you will avoid postpartum charley horse, making this part of your recovery more comfortable.

The eight lower-body exercises in this chapter, as well as the rest of your pregnancy fitness program, will help you have a faster, more comfortable recovery from giving birth and enable you to return quickly to your prepregnancy figure.

FLUTTER KICK

Benefits

Loosens and strengthens the lower back and legs and strengthens the abdominal muscles.

Starting Position

Stand facing the pool wall, at almost arm's length from the edge. Place your hands on the wall with your arms extended and bring your legs toward the water's surface.

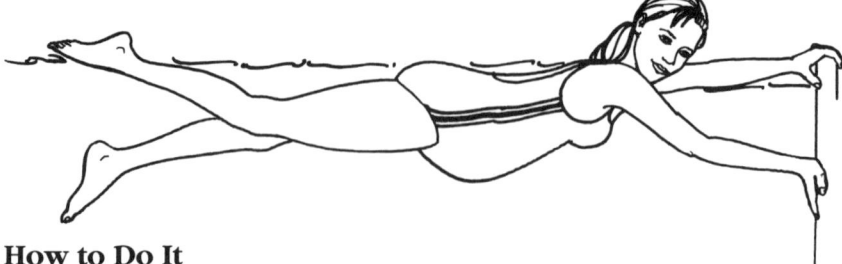

How to Do It

1. Bending your knees slightly and keeping your ankles loose, point your toes inward as you move your legs alternately up and down.
2. Start to kick slowly, then kick progressively faster. As you become more comfortable, you may increase the duration of your kicking exercises.
3. Concentrate on breathing continuously.

Exercise Tips

- Avoid hyperextending your neck and back.
- You may wish to alternate a few seconds of energetic kicking with 5 seconds of easy kicking.

BICYCLE PEDAL

Benefits

Tones the lower body muscles.

Starting Position

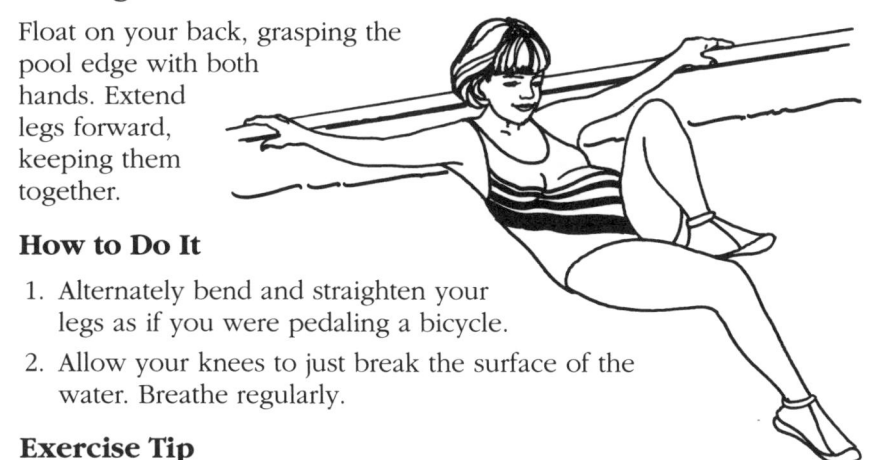

Float on your back, grasping the pool edge with both hands. Extend legs forward, keeping them together.

How to Do It

1. Alternately bend and straighten your legs as if you were pedaling a bicycle.
2. Allow your knees to just break the surface of the water. Breathe regularly.

Exercise Tip

- For extra support, use the corner of the pool, grasping each pool edge. Use extra caution to avoid overstretching the shoulder area. (Joints relax easily during pregnancy.)

Variations

- You can also do this exercise by using a back flutter kick (in which the power comes from hip and thigh muscles) rather than a pedaling motion.
- Another variation is a flutter kick combo: Alternate between the bicycle pedal and flutter kick leg motions.

33

Leg Scissors

Benefits

Stretches the muscles of the abdomen, upper legs, and inner thighs.

Starting Position

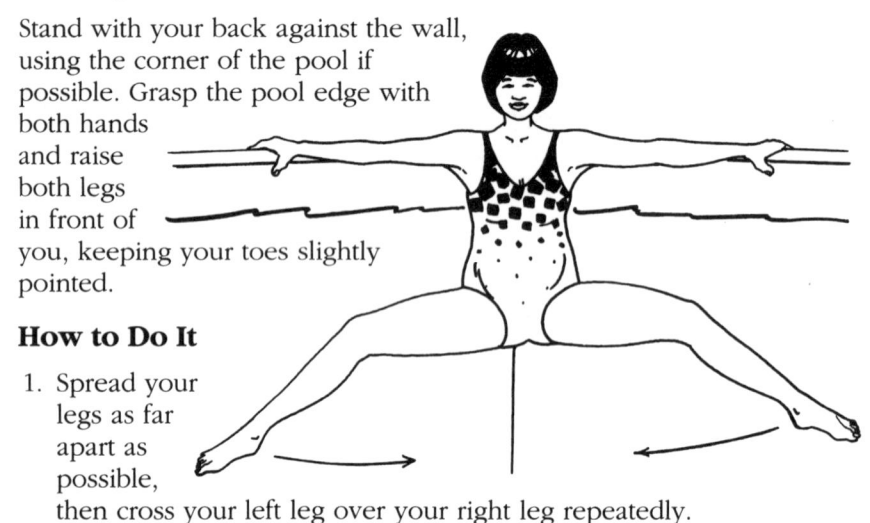

Stand with your back against the wall, using the corner of the pool if possible. Grasp the pool edge with both hands and raise both legs in front of you, keeping your toes slightly pointed.

How to Do It

1. Spread your legs as far apart as possible, then cross your left leg over your right leg repeatedly.
2. Then cross your right leg over your left leg repeatedly.
3. Start with five repetitions per leg and increase the number as you become more comfortable.
4. Remember to breathe regularly by inhaling through your nose and exhaling through your mouth.

Exercise Tips

- Keep your back straight and chin up.
- To help your posture and increase your flexibility, use the pool wall rather than the corner. Use caution to avoid overstretching the shoulder area.

34

CALF STRETCH

Benefits

Stretches and strengthens the calf muscles.

Starting Position

In waist-deep water, stand with legs together on a pool step or a ladder rung. Place your weight on the balls of your feet so that your heels project over the edge. Hold onto the stair or ladder railing for support.

How to Do It

1. Stand on tiptoes and then lower your heels until they are below the ladder or step. Breathe regularly.
2. Return to tiptoes and repeat.

Exercise Tips

- Be sure to maintain supporting grasp on rail.
- For greater buoyancy and support, use lower step on ladder or stairs. For greater resistance and greater weight-bearing effect, use a higher step.

Variation

- If you do not have a safe, comfortable ladder available for your workout, face the pool wall, standing arm's length away. Grasp the edge, step forward with one foot, and shift your weight onto your forward leg, keeping your feet flat on the pool floor. In this lunge position, you will feel the gentle stretch in the calf of your back leg. Then reverse your legs. Try to keep your back leg straight. If the stretch pulls too much, bend your back knee slightly. Keep practicing until your muscles are loosened.

WALL WALK

Benefits

Stretches all the leg muscles, especially those in your thighs, and may help relieve back strain.

Starting Position

Stand in the pool at comfortable depth, facing the pool wall. Grasp the pool edge with both hands.

How to Do It

1. Place your feet flat on the pool wall just above the pool floor.
2. Slowly walk up the wall, no farther than waist level, breathing normally.
3. Then return to a standing position by slowly walking down the pool wall.

Exercise Tip

- Do this exercise only as comfort allows.

Variation

- As your pregnancy progresses, hold onto the pool edge with both feet flat on the pool wall just above the pool bottom. With feet shoulder-width apart, bend and flex your legs.

36

LEG LIFT

Benefits

Stretches and tones your abdomen, lower back, legs, hips, and buttocks.

Starting Position

Stand in the pool in waist-deep water, legs together, with your back against the pool wall; hold onto the edge with both hands and forearms.

How to Do It

1. Raise one leg in front of you as high as you can comfortably. Keep your hips against the wall.
2. Then lower your leg. Do the same number of repetitions for each leg.
3. Breathe in through your nose each time you raise your leg and out through your mouth each time you lower your leg. Breathe continuously.

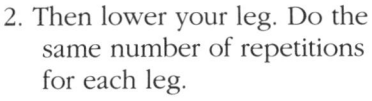

Exercise Tips

- Keep your leg as straight as is comfortable (a "soft" knee) without locking your knee.
- Do not point your toes.

37

Leg Swirl

Benefits

Strengthens and tones lower abdominal and leg muscles.

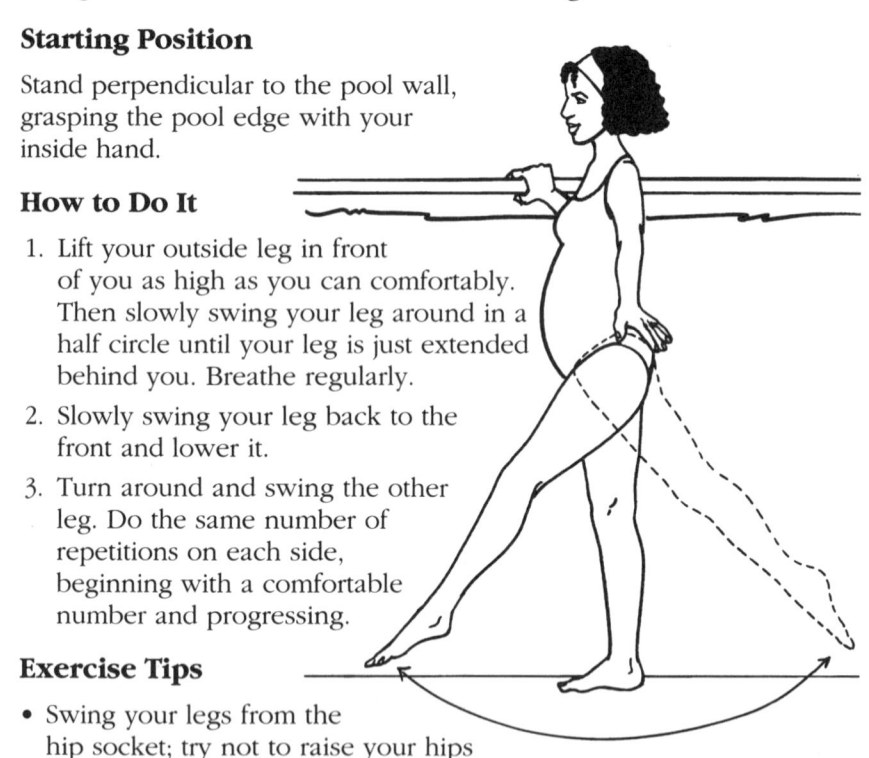

Starting Position

Stand perpendicular to the pool wall, grasping the pool edge with your inside hand.

How to Do It

1. Lift your outside leg in front of you as high as you can comfortably. Then slowly swing your leg around in a half circle until your leg is just extended behind you. Breathe regularly.
2. Slowly swing your leg back to the front and lower it.
3. Turn around and swing the other leg. Do the same number of repetitions on each side, beginning with a comfortable number and progressing.

Exercise Tips

- Swing your legs from the hip socket; try not to raise your hips from their normal position.
- Retain good posture and body alignment.

Variations

- Foot Circles: Stand perpendicular to the pool wall, grasping the pool edge with your inside hand. Lift your outside leg in front of you and trace a small circle in the water with your foot in a clockwise direction. Follow this by tracing a circle in a counterclockwise direction. Do the same number of repetitions of each movement for each leg. You can also "write" names, numbers, and so on in the water.
- Stand with back against the wall in a pelvic tilt position and modify exercise to comfort level.

38

DOUBLE LEG CIRCLE

Benefits

Strengthens your abdominal muscles and stretches inner-thigh muscles. This exercise is ideal for maintaining proper posture.

Starting Position

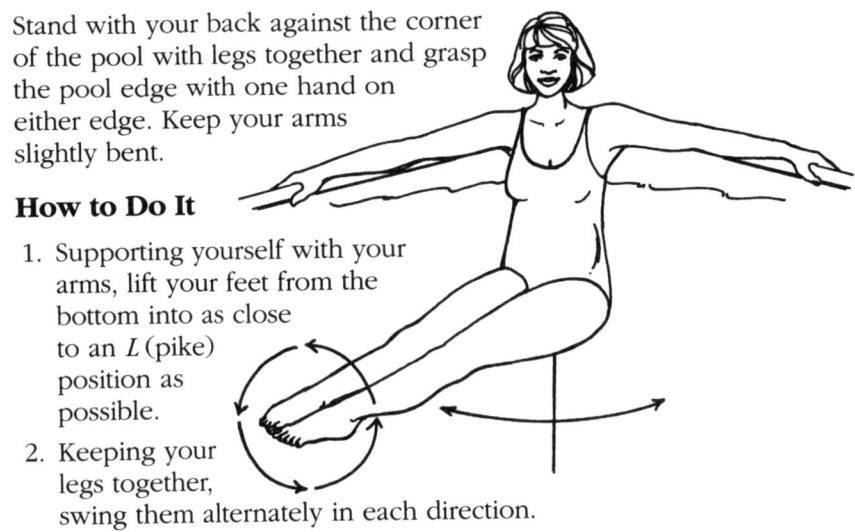

Stand with your back against the corner of the pool with legs together and grasp the pool edge with one hand on either edge. Keep your arms slightly bent.

How to Do It

1. Supporting yourself with your arms, lift your feet from the bottom into as close to an *L* (pike) position as possible.
2. Keeping your legs together, swing them alternately in each direction.
3. "Draw" circles with your legs together. Then reverse the directions of the circles. Do the same number of repetitions in each direction. Breathe regularly.
4. End this exercise by bringing your legs down to the pool floor and touching your heels together, bending your knees outward. This stretches your inner-thigh muscles.

Exercise Tips

- If you feel undue strain in your back, do not do this exercise.
- Use extra caution to avoid overstretching the shoulder area.

Variations

- Try the Double Leg Circle with your feet flexed—this will change the stretch.
- If you find these exercises becoming too difficult as your pregnancy progresses, do them sitting at the edge of the pool.

chapter 8

TOTAL-BODY EXERCISES

We have just highlighted over two dozen exercises for the large muscle groups of the upper, middle, and lower body and for the intercostal muscles (between your ribs). Each of these exercise groups focuses on a particular area, but many water exercises combine more than one body area. These are called total-body exercises. Just as you have several concerns simultaneously during pregnancy, so these water exercises tone and stretch several areas of your body at once.

The five total-body exercises give you practice in body coordination, which may help you during labor and delivery, especially if you have not been involved in some kind of physical activity before your pregnancy. They also improve your conditioning.

39

ARM AND LEG REACH

Benefits

Tones and stretches the entire body, especially the trunk, arm, and upper-leg muscles.

Equipment

Fins (optional)

Starting Position

Stand in chest-deep water, perpendicular to the pool wall, with legs comfortably together. Hold onto the pool edge and lean forward slightly.

How to Do It

1. Extend your outside arm forward and upward as you bend your outside knee to bring your foot behind you.
2. Then reach back with your outside arm and grasp your ankle, stretching your thigh muscles.
3. Release your ankle and slowly return to the starting position. Repeat exercise on your other side by turning around.
4. Inhale slowly through your nose as you grasp your ankle and stretch, and exhale slowly through your mouth as you release and return.

Exercise Tip

- If it is difficult for you to reach your foot, you can wear fins to "lengthen" your feet.

Total-Body Exercises 77

40

PENDULUM BODY SWING

Benefits

Tones and stretches the muscles of your entire body, especially at your sides, which are often overlooked.

Starting Position

Stand with legs together in neck-deep water with your back against the pool wall.

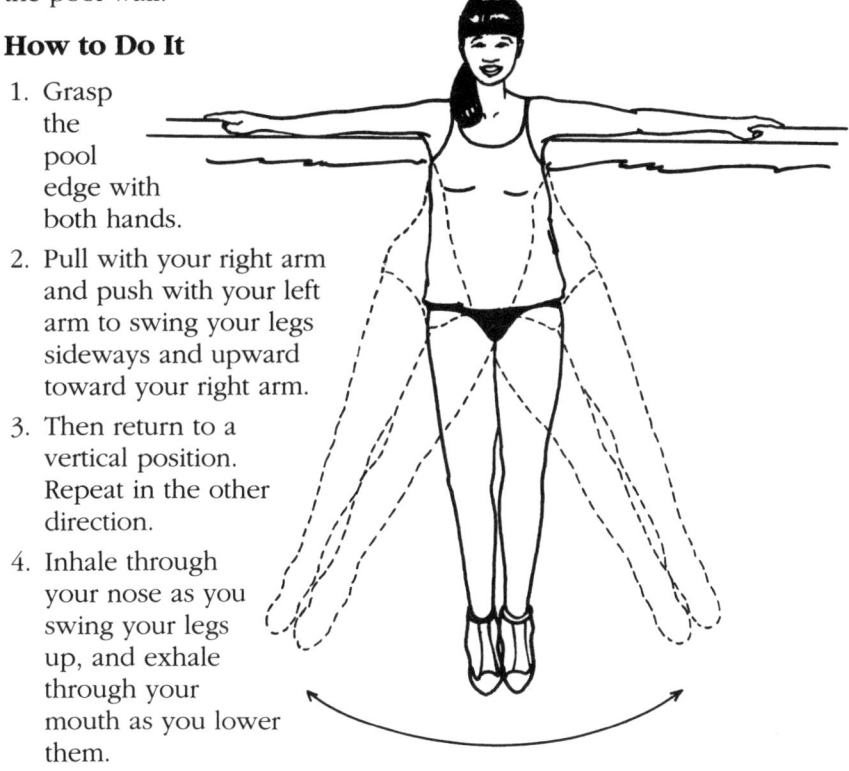

How to Do It

1. Grasp the pool edge with both hands.
2. Pull with your right arm and push with your left arm to swing your legs sideways and upward toward your right arm.
3. Then return to a vertical position. Repeat in the other direction.
4. Inhale through your nose as you swing your legs up, and exhale through your mouth as you lower them.

Exercise Tips

- If swinging both legs is too difficult, begin with one leg at a time.
- Use extra caution to avoid overstretching the shoulder area.

41

TREADING

Benefits
Overall conditioning.

Equipment
Flotation support

Starting Position
Stand in neck-deep water, feet just touching bottom.

How to Do It

1. Lean forward slightly in the water and bend your knees. Bring your legs up from the pool bottom by beginning a "bicycle" leg motion.
2. Add a wide, slow sculling figure-eight arm motion.
3. Vary the direction in which you travel through the water, using forward, backward, sideways, and circular routes.
4. Breathe continuously and deeply, inhaling through your nose and exhaling through your mouth.
5. If you are not an experienced swimmer, use a flotation device to help support yourself.

Exercise Tips

- Relaxed, slow treading movements are the most effective.
- Treading is not only a total-body exercise, it is also a deep-water safety skill.
- Try different leg variations for treading, including the bicycle leg motion, frog kick, and scissors kick.

Variation

- Eggbeater Kick: In this more energetic variation each leg moves alternately, circling inward. This kick is often used in synchronized swimming or lifesaving. (The leg movements are similar to the spokes of an eggbeater.)

Posture Check

Benefits

Helps in body alignment, which is a major factor in comfort during your pregnancy, and relieves strain on back muscles.

Starting Position

Stand in chest-deep water with feet together and soft knees, with your shoulders, back, buttocks, and heels against the pool wall. Grasp the pool edge with both hands for support. The small of your back should be against the wall.

How to Do It

1. Bend your knees and place your feet flat against the pool wall, supporting yourself. Keep your arms straight. Breathe regularly.
2. Hold for a count of 10, then rest.

Exercise Tip

- Try to keep your back against the wall to ease lower-back stress.

Variation

- You can also practice a variation of this exercise at home. Lie on the floor with your knees bent and your feet flat on the floor, as close to your buttocks as possible. Lift your hips off the floor, so that your body is straight from your knees to your chest. Inhale through your nose as you lift your hips and exhale through your mouth as you lower your legs.

43

DEEP-WATER JOG

Benefits

Allows you to practice running coordination for overall conditioning without impact and/or risk of injury. (Runners and joggers especially enjoy deep-water jogging.)

Equipment

Flotation support such as a belt or buoyancy vest. Be sure it fits comfortably and does not press on your abdomen.

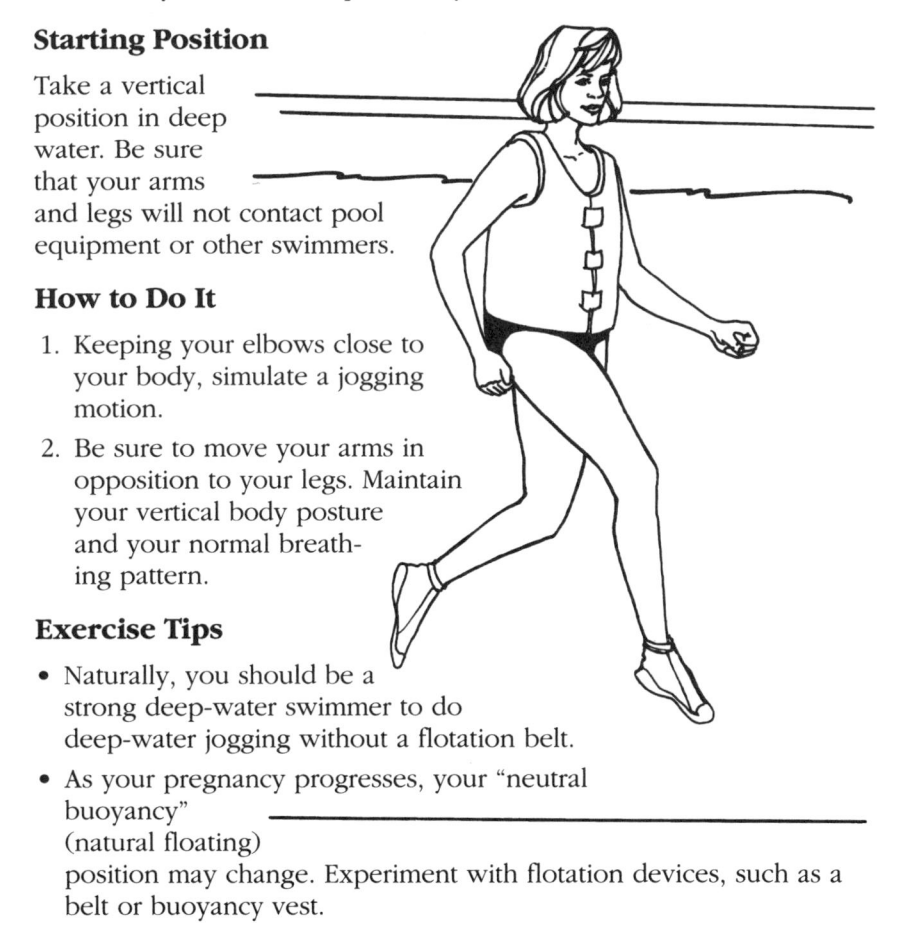

Starting Position

Take a vertical position in deep water. Be sure that your arms and legs will not contact pool equipment or other swimmers.

How to Do It

1. Keeping your elbows close to your body, simulate a jogging motion.
2. Be sure to move your arms in opposition to your legs. Maintain your vertical body posture and your normal breathing pattern.

Exercise Tips

- Naturally, you should be a strong deep-water swimmer to do deep-water jogging without a flotation belt.
- As your pregnancy progresses, your "neutral buoyancy" (natural floating) position may change. Experiment with flotation devices, such as a belt or buoyancy vest.

- As your pregnancy advances, deep-water jogging may not work for you. You may be more comfortable treading, using an eggbeater kick.
- Vary your Deep-Water Jog by simulating cross-country skiing, with your arms and legs moving in opposition. Aim for increased range of motion, forward and back; keep your range of motion as extended and equidistant as possible.

part III

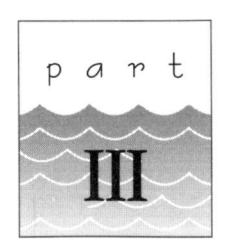

SWIM STROKES

Swimming is a skill with a scientific base. Whether you swim for recreation, do fitness laps, or swim at the Master level, the following chapters will help you improve your swim stroke technique. Each chapter includes skills to help you master specific stroke techniques, especially those that make the difference between average and above-average swimming.

Your decision to swim for fitness during your pregnancy is an excellent one because pregnancy limits your fitness choices. A swim workout gives you a mental respite from daily activities—you don't have to answer phone calls when you're under the water! With common sense and a little knowledge, you can make your swim workout refreshing and invigorating.

First let's look at the scientific principles that are the basis for good swim skills:

- *Buoyancy*. The specific gravity of water is 1.0. Because your specific gravity is less, you will float. As your pregnancy advances, your specific gravity will decrease, and you'll become more buoyant.
- *Center of gravity*. Proper body position is essential for everyday activities. It is particularly important for you now because your center of gravity will shift as your pregnancy progresses and you may tend to lose your balance more easily. However, a little caution goes a long way toward fitness safety.

This shift in your center of gravity also puts added pressure on areas of your body that may not otherwise be subject to strain. This pressure frequently causes muscle discomfort. The buoyancy of the water, however, supports and cushions the body, relieving strain. That is one reason swimming is so relaxing during pregnancy.

- *Newton's third law of motion.* Simply stated, for every action, there is an equal and opposite reaction. That is, when you push your arm against the water (pushing water behind you), you propel yourself in the opposite direction—forward.

The chapters that follow will discuss these components for each stroke:

1. *Body position.* All strokes begin and maintain a specific body position. Position is important for comfort and relaxation as well as for better stroke coordination.
2. *Arm motion.* Although arm strokes vary, they all share the following elements:
   - *The catch*, the starting point of your hand and arm in the water.
   - *The pull*, the propulsion stage during which you push water backward in order to go forward.
   - *The recovery*, the resting stage during which you return your arm to the catch position.
3. *Leg motion.* For each of the strokes, you use your hip, thigh, and leg muscles during the kick to complement the forward effect of the arm motion.
4. *Breathing.* Good breathing skills are necessary to provide you with sufficient oxygen for your swim workout.
5. *Stroke coordination.* Coordinating all these components with breathing in each stroke produces smooth, fluid movement.

In addition to stroke components, these chapters include descriptions of appropriate push-offs and turns, tips for swimming during pregnancy, illustrations of each stroke, and two exercises to reinforce stroke skills. Chapter 9 covers the crawl stroke, chapter 10 reviews the breaststroke, chapter 11 contains three forms of the backstroke, and chapter 12 covers the relaxing sidestroke.

Although this part of *Water Fitness During Your Pregnancy* reviews the components of swimming, this is not a learn-to-swim manual. Instead it is an opportunity to review strokes you have learned previously so you can swim better and derive the greatest benefit from your water fitness workouts during your pregnancy.

chapter 9

CRAWL STROKE

All swim strokes begin in a horizontal body position—swimming literally and figuratively gives you a lift because you're off your feet. And because the buoyancy of the water supports your weight, water activities are comfortable fitness alternatives.

This chapter highlights each component of the crawl stroke with an exercise to reinforce your stroke skill. These drills for both arms and legs also help develop the strength and overall body tone that you'll need during and after your pregnancy. The crawl stroke is especially beneficial for developing upper-body conditioning.

Research has found that the better condition you are in, the happier and healthier your pregnancy is likely to be. Exercising gives you a psychological boost so you'll have more energy throughout the day for your home, work, and your other children. Let's start!

The Stroke

The crawl stroke is perhaps the first stroke you learned. When most North Americans think about swimming, they think about the crawl stroke. Maybe it is the easiest stroke to learn because the opposing arm and leg motions are similar to walking. The leverage of the arm stroke works efficiently to draw your body through the water. This gives the crawl stroke most of its speed.

Body Position

Your body is prone (face down) in the water forming a long streamlined shape along your central axis (your spine). The water level should come between your eyebrows and your hairline.

Arm Motion

The arm motion consists of three parts: the *catch*, the *pull*, and the *recovery*. One stroke of each arm including the catch, pull, and recovery make up an arm cycle.

The *catch* begins each stroke with your hand slicing into the water fingertips first and moving to a position 6 to 8 inches under the water's surface at a 30° to 40° angle (see Figure 9.1). Your arm then is extended fully into the water. The *pull* begins by pressing the water downward, but mostly backward toward your thighs, bending your arm as you pull and keeping your hand close to your thigh at the end of the stroke. This *pull* is what propels you through the water. The recovery follows as your arm lifts out of the water and returns to the starting catch position. Keep your elbow higher than your hand during the recovery.

Leg Motion

The crawl stroke uses the flutter kick; your legs move up and down as if you were walking. The action of the kick comes from your hips and thighs. Your knees should be slightly flexed, but your ankles should be loose and relaxed for comfort and efficiency. Rather than overkicking and splashing, you should just make the water "boil." The kick is used primarily to stabilize your stroke and body position. As your pregnancy advances, you will find your body position changes—as you inhale and turn your head to one side for breathing you may need to use a crossover kick or a variation of a scissors kick (see p. 115).

Breathing

The correct way to get air continuously while doing the crawl is through rhythmic breathing. Once you know this technique, you'll agree that using it is really the easiest way to swim the crawl stroke.

You will probably have a definite preference as to whether you turn your head to the right or to the left during rhythmic breathing. Choose the side that is most comfortable for you, and then continue to use that side. (The only exception is for serious fitness swimmers who use alternate breathing, turning for a breath on every third arm stroke rather than every other arm stroke.)

Rhythmic breathing is done by turning your face to one side out of the water to inhale, and then turning back into the water to exhale. Exhale completely—you should form bubbles in the water. Use both your nose and mouth for inhaling and exhaling. Not breathing properly will cause you to tire easily. (See the breathing exercises in chapter 4.)

Stroke Coordination

To breathe rhythmically and coordinate the arm motion of the stroke, follow the law of opposites: As you turn your head to one side to inhale, extend your arm forward on the opposite or nonbreathing side, with your

Crawl Stroke **87**

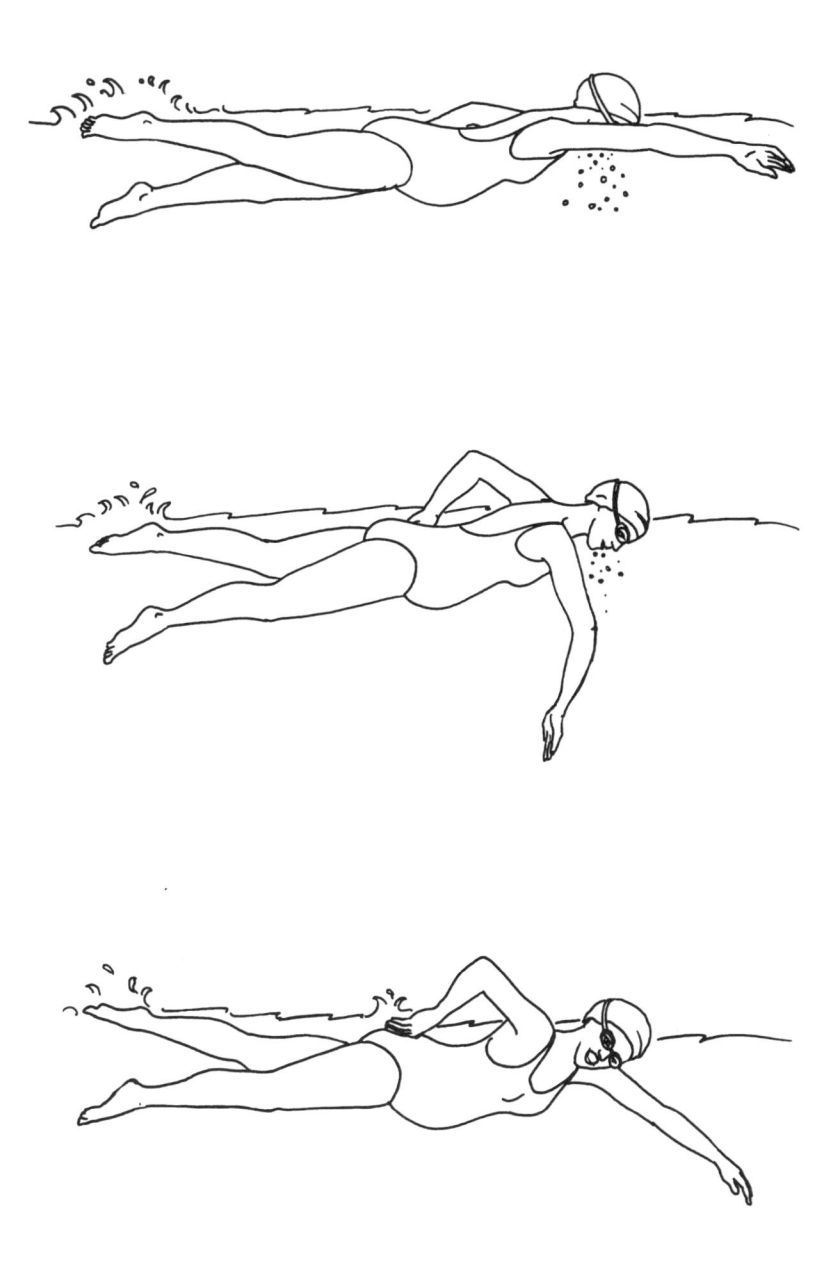

Figure 9.1 The crawl stroke arm motion.

hand gliding into the water. Keep the arm on your breathing side back and ready to recover. Continue the *pull* of the opposite arm as you inhale, and then pivot your head so that your face is back in the water. Begin exhaling immediately. At the same time, your arm on your breathing side finishes its recovery.

Crawl Stroke Refinements

You may have heard the word *freestyle* used interchangeably with *crawl stroke*, but there is a distinction. The freestyle adds a number of stroke refinements to the crawl to make it faster and more efficient. Used together, these techniques improve your swimming and are helpful during pregnancy because they strengthen your upper body and add variety and interest to your workout.

S-Shaped Pull

The S-shaped pull displaces still water rather than water that has already been set in motion, enabling you to move a greater volume of water with each stroke and propelling you farther forward.

The S-shaped pull consists of two parts. For the first part, start at the *catch* position and trace a reverse *S* (or a question mark) with your right hand by pulling outward (away from the center of your body) and downward (toward the pool bottom; see Figure 9.2). As your hand passes your head, begin pulling inward toward your waist. In the second part, press your hand back, moving it diagonally toward your thigh. Straighten and extend your arm as you accelerate your movement.

For your left arm, trace a letter *S* or a reverse question mark using the same motions.

Body Roll

As each arm recovers, the body has a natural tendency to roll almost 45° toward the arm that is pulling. Don't resist this action; it has advantages. Because of the body roll, your shoulder and back muscles provide increased leverage to your pulling arm, which strengthens your pull. Also this body roll makes it easier to turn your head to take a breath. However, you should not roll more than 45°.

Crossover Kick

As each shoulder follows your arm into the water with the S-shaped pull, your hips naturally follow the roll of your shoulder. This results in your feet crossing at the lower part of the leg. To optimize this motion, modify the flutter kick to help balance your body in the water. As your right shoulder rolls downward and the arm pulls, dip your right hip down and cross the left foot behind the right foot. For the left-arm pull, do the opposite. The crossover kick gives your freestyle a smooth, even cadence.

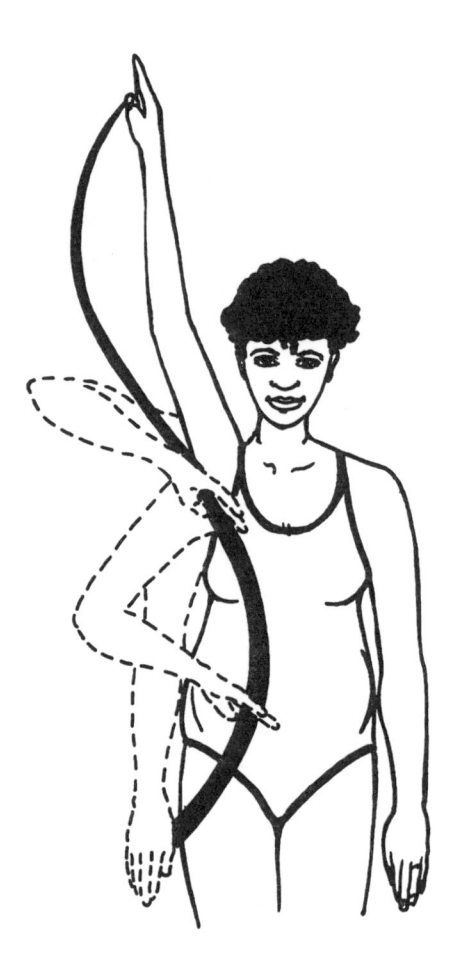

Figure 9.2 The S-shaped pull variation.

Push-Off

During your pregnancy, safety is the first consideration in water fitness. Although it may seem repetitious to continue to emphasize this, your peace of mind is well worth the precautions you take. So during your pregnancy, forceful entries into the water, whether diving or jumping, are *not* recommended. Enter the pool carefully using the stairs or ladder, or slide slowly into the pool from a sitting position.

To begin a lap, stand in the water with your knees slightly bent, your back foot against the wall, and your arms extended in front of you in a streamlined position (see Figure 9.3). Lower your body underwater, place your other foot against the wall, and push both legs into a glide. Your legs provide the power for the push-off, and the resistance of the pool wall or bottom helps make it efficient. During the push-off, align your head with

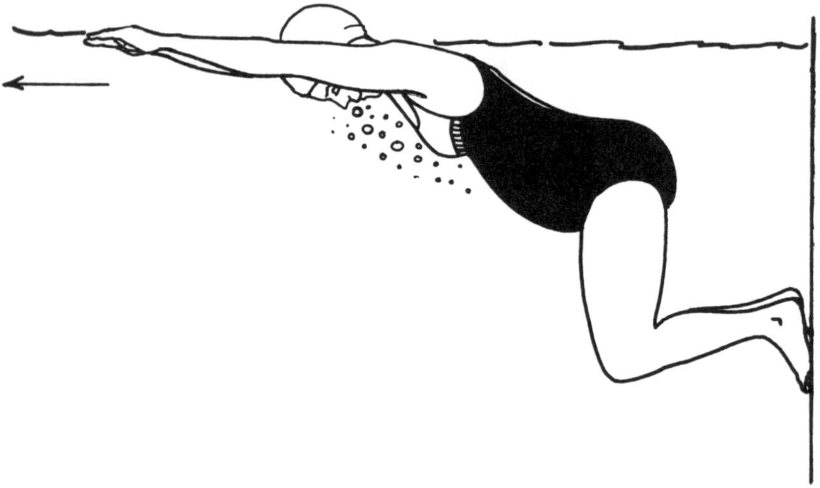

Figure 9.3 The crawl stroke push-off.

your body. Keep your arms overhead, covering your ears during the glide, and streamline your body. Begin your crawl stroke when your glide begins to lose momentum.

As your pregnancy advances, you will become more buoyant. To help counteract the tendency to "pop up" in the water during your crawl push-off, lower your head and angle your arms under the water toward the bottom of the pool. You can use the sidestroke push-off (see p. 116) as a variation of the crawl starting position if it is more comfortable as your pregnancy progresses.

The effect of pushing off helps strengthen and condition your legs. The longer you hold your streamlined glide position during your push-off, the more it will help stretch leg muscles. Always push off gently—your ligaments are softened during pregnancy (in preparation for birth), so you are more prone to injury without being aware of it.

Turn

The purpose of a turn is to use the body's momentum to make a 180° rotation, from one direction to the opposite direction. During pregnancy it is recommended that you use an open turn. If you are a fitness swimmer and accustomed to flip turns, use them only as long as you are comfortable; pregnancy isn't time to prove your grit. Your comfort and the safety of your baby are of utmost importance. If you haven't been using flip turns, wait until you're fully recovered after your baby is born to try them. Then learning a flip turn can be your short-term recovery project.

For an open turn, swim toward the pool wall with your eyes open, looking forward so you can see the marker. When you are about a body length from the wall, complete your arm stroke and continue kicking to the wall with one arm extended. Turn your other arm in the direction in which you will be turning. As your forward hand touches the wall, bend your elbow to bring your body close to the wall, keeping your head out of the water (see Figure 9.4). Bend your knees under your body and turn away from your forward hand. As you rotate, place your feet on the wall and stretch out your arms in the direction in which you will be swimming. With both knees bent, gently straighten your legs for the push-off.

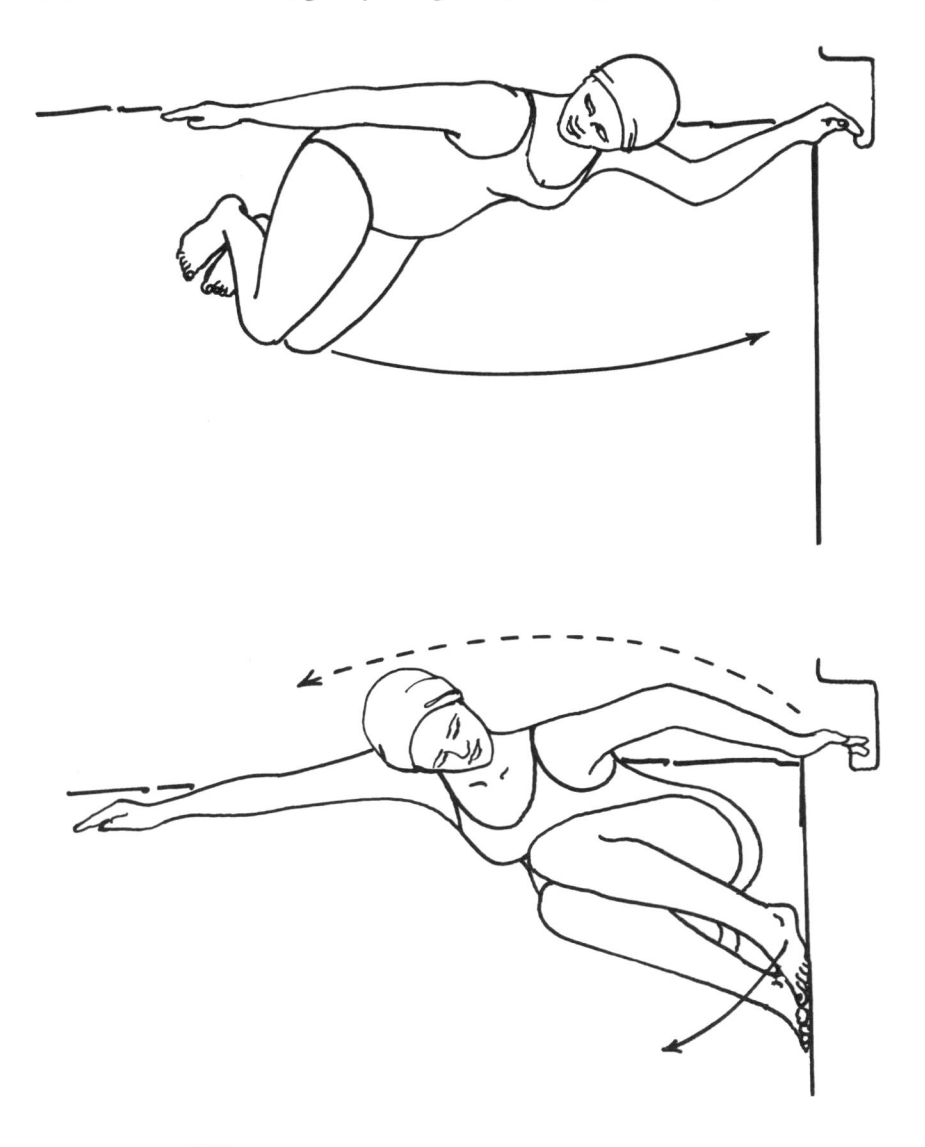

Figure 9.4 The crawl stroke open turn.

Crawl Stroke Tips

- Maintain your streamlined body position as you swim.
- To get the most from each arm motion, stretch your arm out on the catch and complete the pull to your hip.
- In order to pull through the water effectively, keep your hand and forearm at a fixed angle, with your thumb and fingertips entering the water during the catch and pull.
- Keep your elbows higher than your hands during recovery.
- Remember not to overkick. It will tire you out unnecessarily and be uncomfortable. Adjust your kick so the water at your feet appears to "boil."
- If you feel out of breath, stop and rest. (Think safety!) You may want to review your rhythmic breathing technique to be sure your air exchange is complete. Avoid hyperventilation—taking in more oxygen than you need.
- When inhaling, rotate your head so your nose and mouth just clear the water.
- Use the nose and mouth to inhale and to exhale. Don't forget to exhale fully. Breathe continuously. (Being conscious of your breathing is good practice for labor and delivery breathing.)
- If you are an advanced swimmer familiar with alternate breathing, use it as a variation of rhythmic breathing. Turn for a breath on every third arm stroke, rather than on your second arm stroke. This helps develop breathing capacity. Use it as far into your pregnancy as you are comfortable.
- Listen to your body—rest when you need to.

44

RHYTHMIC BREATHING

Benefits

Practices the rhythmic breathing technique for the crawl stroke.

Starting Position

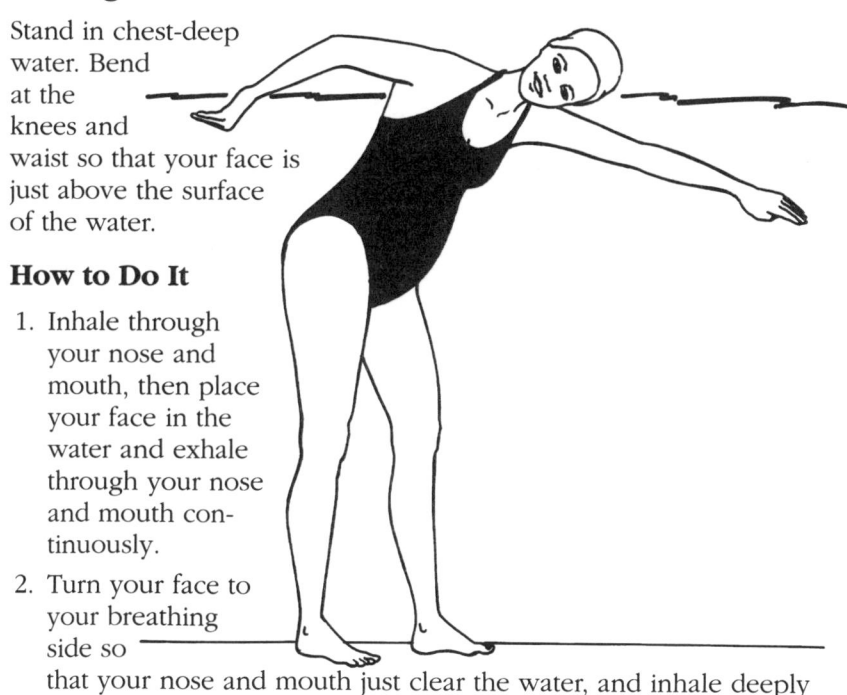

Stand in chest-deep water. Bend at the knees and waist so that your face is just above the surface of the water.

How to Do It

1. Inhale through your nose and mouth, then place your face in the water and exhale through your nose and mouth continuously.
2. Turn your face to your breathing side so that your nose and mouth just clear the water, and inhale deeply through your nose and mouth.
3. Turn your face back into the water and exhale through your nose and mouth, forming bubbles. Repeat 5 to 10 times, rest, and then repeat.

Variation

- You can practice coordinating your breathing with your arm stroke by doing the "walking crawl." Stand, then walk forward as you perform the arm stroke and rhythmic breathing. Remember that as one hand extends forward to stroke and the other recovers, you turn your face to the side of the recovering hand to breathe.

45

Catch-Up Arm Stroke

Benefits

Helps isolate the S-shaped pull for more efficient swimming.

Equipment

Kickboard

Starting Position

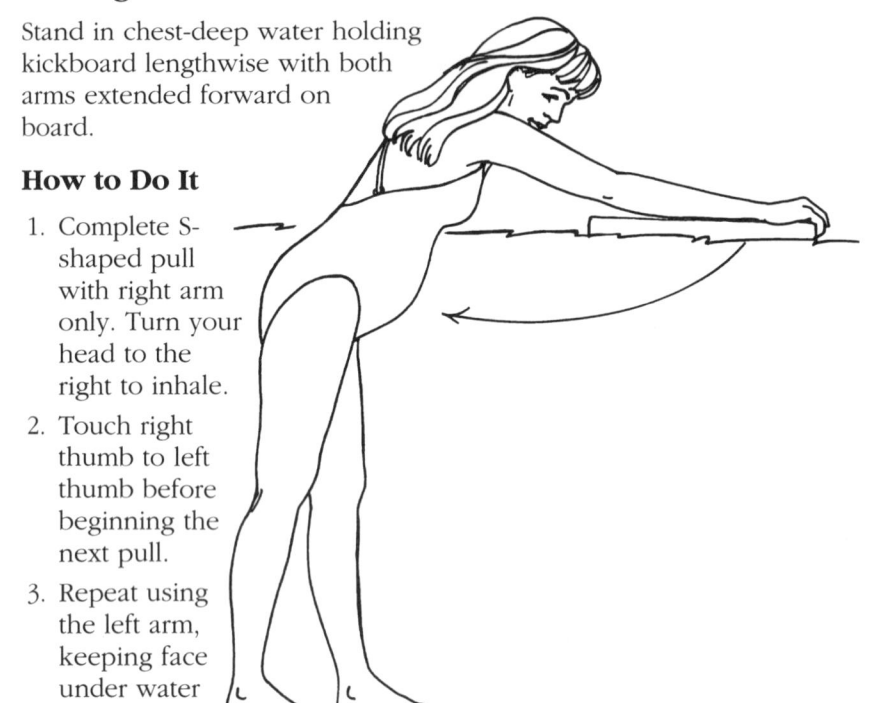

Stand in chest-deep water holding kickboard lengthwise with both arms extended forward on board.

How to Do It

1. Complete S-shaped pull with right arm only. Turn your head to the right to inhale.
2. Touch right thumb to left thumb before beginning the next pull.
3. Repeat using the left arm, keeping face under water to exhale.

Exercise Tips

- Slow down pull arm motion as much as possible.
- Feel your arm pushing the water behind you in the S-shaped pattern.

Variation

- Walk forward using the S-shaped pull.

chapter 10

BREASTSTROKE

Historically, the breaststroke is the oldest stroke. If your family is from Europe, this may have been the first stroke you learned.

Although you should wear goggles during your lap swim workout, the breaststroke is a good stroke to choose if you decide not to wear them. If you will be using the breaststroke, you may need to swim in a slower lane than you are accustomed to. Just as you are careful to avoid other swimmers to prevent injury to you and your baby, be careful where you swim while doing the breaststroke so you won't accidentally collide with someone else in the pool.

This chapter, like the preceding chapter on the crawl, includes stroke skills and coordination, information on turns and push-offs, stroke tips, and skill-specific drills.

The Stroke

Breaststroke is an easy and relaxing stroke when you swim slowly. The heart-shaped circular arm motion and the kick provide equal propulsion. The breaststroke is an excellent way to vary the pace of your swim workout.

Breaststroke is recommended throughout your pregnancy. This stroke coordinates your breathing with your armstroke because your head rises with your shoulders, affording you a good view. The arms and legs each provide the same amount of forward propulsion. Breaststroke movements are especially helpful in toning and stretching leg muscles. The breaststroke's long and restful glide makes it ideal for the last months of your pregnancy.

Body Position

Extend your body in the prone (face-down) position. At the beginning of your stroke (glide position), extend your arms straight in front of you, with your feet just below the surface. Always look in the direction you are swimming.

Arm Motion

In the breaststroke, your arms move simultaneously and symmetrically under the water during the entire stroke. As your arms move together they trace the outline of a heart during the pull phase of the arm motion. On the recovery, both arms are extended straight ahead under the water.

The *catch* begins with your hands about as far apart as your shoulders. Rotate your wrists so your palms face outward with your thumbs pointing downward, allowing your hands to get a hold on the water. During the *pull* keep your elbows higher than your hands. The most efficient pull ends approximately at your shoulders. The *recovery* should be a smooth, natural motion that immediately follows. Recover with your palms close together in a prayer position. *Glide* with your arms extended before the next stroke.

Leg Motion

Two kicks are commonly used in the breaststroke. Most people know the *frog kick*. Fitness and competitive swimmers use a *whip kick* or a *modified whip kick*. If you do either of these kicks now, it is fine to continue as long as you are comfortable.

The *frog kick* is especially good during pregnancy because it exercises the legs, hips, and thighs while you are prone in the water. Spread your knees wider than your hips and drop them slightly as you bring your heels together. Then extend your legs by straightening them at the knees while flexing your feet so your legs form a wide *V*. Bring your legs (which should be straight at this point) together while pointing your toes to complete the kick. The *whip kick* is similar to the frog kick, except that the knees are closer together, within the width of the hips. In the *modified whip kick*, the knees are farther apart than in the *whip kick*, but not as far apart as in the *frog kick*.

Breathing

Inhale as your head and shoulders rise when you widen your arm pull; exhale as your face submerges and your arms recover to the glide position.

Stroke Coordination

The basic stroke sequence is pull (inhale), kick, recover, and glide (exhale). To coordinate the breaststroke, begin the pull first and follow with the kick. Bend your knees to begin the kick, then continue both arm and leg motions simultaneously to finish the stroke, with your body fully extended and streamlined for the glide (see Figure 10.1).

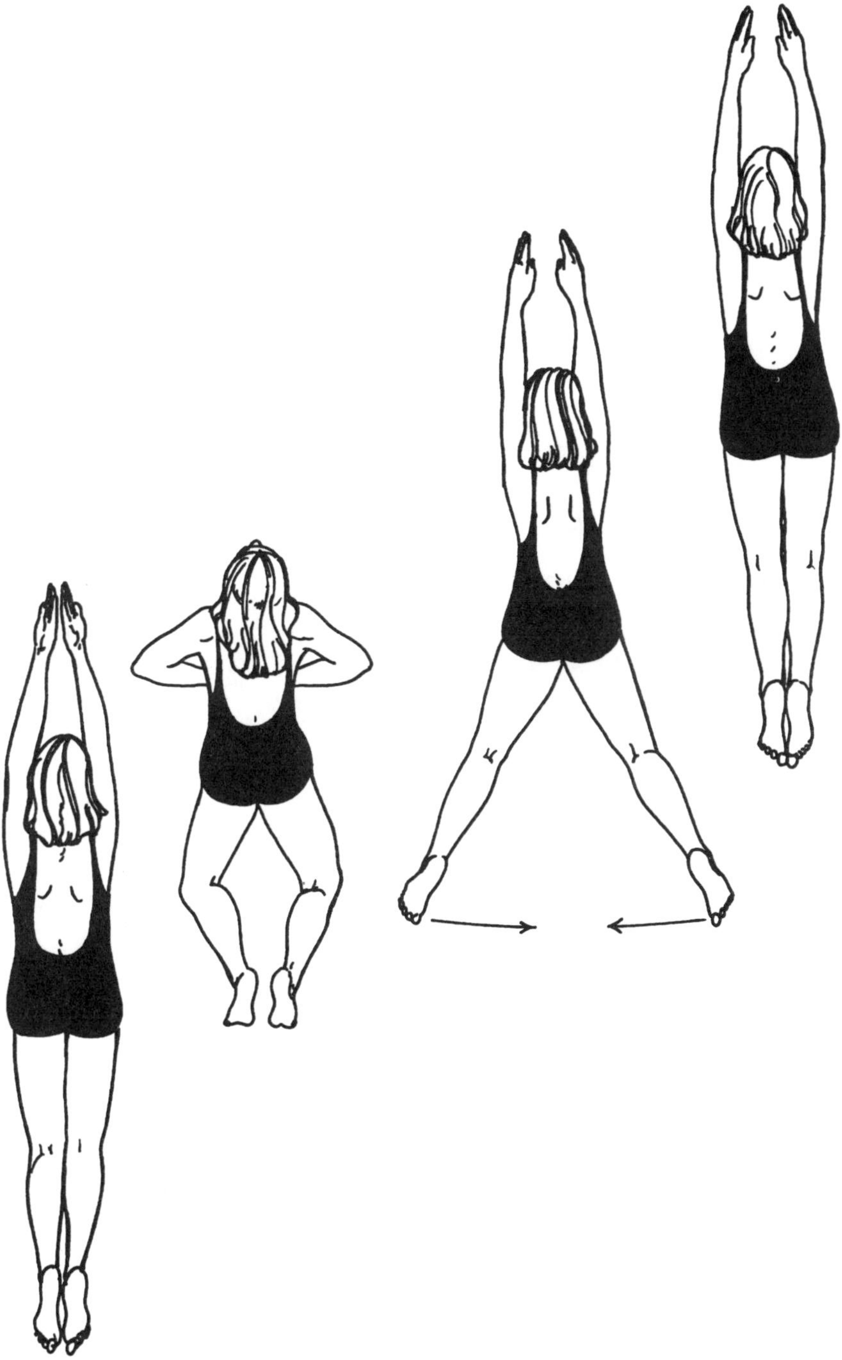

Figure 10.1 The breaststroke arm motion and stroke coordination.

Push-Off

Stand against the wall with your knees slightly bent, one foot against the wall, and your arms extended in front of you in a streamlined position. Lower your body underwater while bringing your other foot onto the wall, and push with both legs into a glide.

It might be helpful to push off at a downward angle toward the pool bottom with your hips higher than your head and arms—this is known as downstreaming. You'll feel as if you're going downhill for a moment, but this will give you more glide.

Turn

The breaststroke turn is similar to the crawl turn, with minor differences because of the breaststroke's symmetrical motion. As you approach the wall at the end of each lap, touch the pool edge with both hands. Turn in either direction, release the wall with either arm, and push off.

Breaststroke Tips

- You have a better view when you use this stroke because you are always looking forward. You can feel more relaxed and confident because you know where you are in relation to other swimmers.
- The heart-shaped pull involves pulling your arms wide toward shoulder width, keeping your elbows higher than your hands.
- Inhale when your head and shoulders rise naturally above the water as a result of your pull.
- Be as streamlined and relaxed as possible during the glide.
- To stretch and tone your upper body, emphasize the heart-shaped arm motion.
- The frog kick, like a cross-legged sitting position, helps stretch inner thigh muscles, which is helpful as you approach your delivery date.
- Differences in horizontal buoyancy are based on many variables, such as body build and baby weight. You might find yourself swimming lower in the water as your pregnancy progresses.
- Also as your pregnancy progresses, you might find it more comfortable to return to a frog kick from a whip kick.
- Also as your pregnancy progresses, your feet may break the surface more often than before. If they do, try dropping your knees farther down before extending them into the *V* position.

46

BREASTSTROKE ARM PULL

Benefits

Provides practice for the heart-shaped breaststroke pull while strengthening the pectoral muscles for chest support.

Starting Position

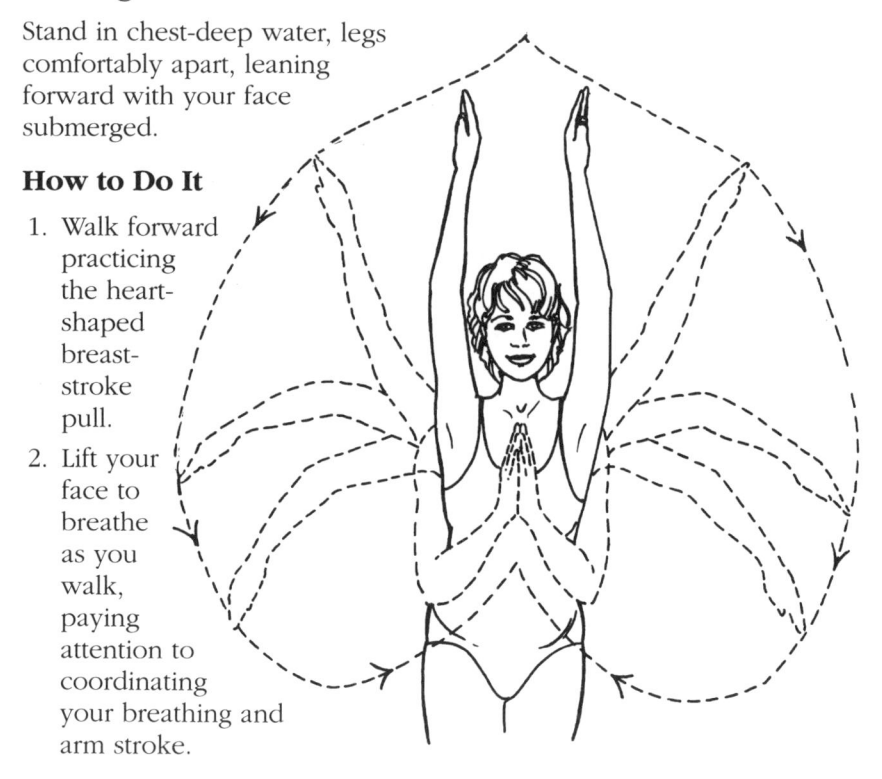

Stand in chest-deep water, legs comfortably apart, leaning forward with your face submerged.

How to Do It

1. Walk forward practicing the heart-shaped breaststroke pull.
2. Lift your face to breathe as you walk, paying attention to coordinating your breathing and arm stroke.

Exercise Tip

- While swimming breaststroke laps, count the number of arm strokes you need to complete a lap. On succeeding laps, try to decrease this number.

FROG KICK

Benefits

Gives you a chance to practice your breaststroke kick and to tone and strengthen your leg muscles. This kick also stretches your inner thigh muscles.

Equipment

Kickboard (optional)

Starting Position

Stand facing the pool wall, at almost arm's distance from the edge.

How to Do It

1. Hold onto the wall in bracket position (see p. 58). Bring your body to prone-float position.
2. Practice your frog kick. Concentrate on streamlined and graceful form.
3. Breathe rhythmically by inhaling out of the water and exhaling under the water.

Exercise Tip

- Avoid jerky motions.

Variations

- Practice your frog kick using a kickboard by extending your arms straight in front of you and grasping the kickboard. Either keep your head above water and breathe normally or coordinate inhalation and exhalation with the kick.
- While supporting yourself in the water with a figure-eight arm scull (p. 52), do the frog kick in a vertical position.

Breaststroke 101

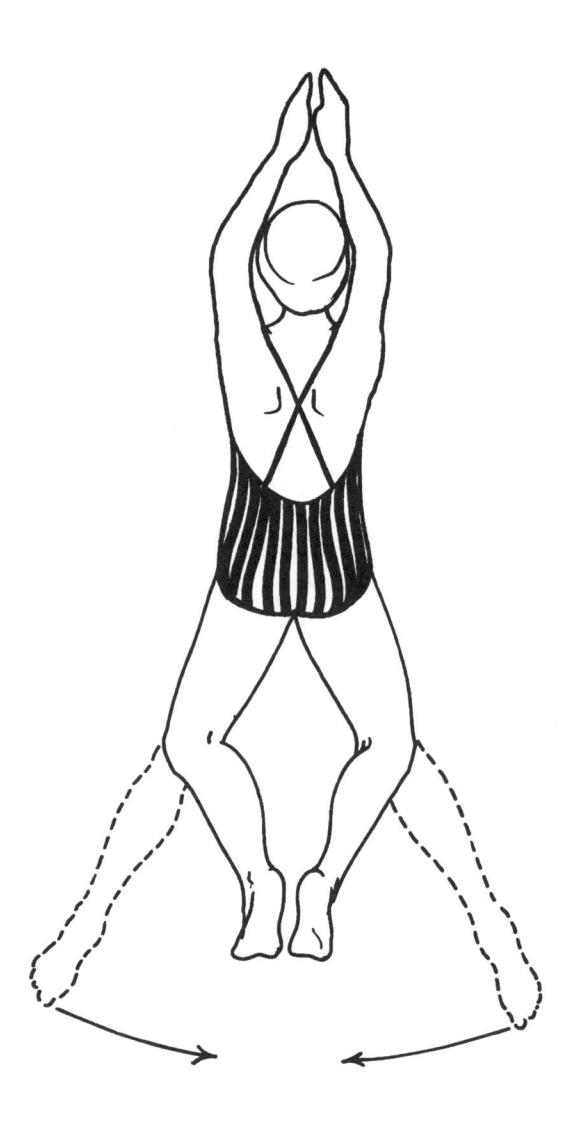

chapter 11

BACKSTROKE

Many swimmers enjoy the backstroke because it leaves the face out of the water. Breathing during this stroke is comfortable. Because you're swimming on your back and your nose and mouth are exposed, breathing is more natural. Some people enjoy the backstroke because they can see what is happening around them.

Backstroke has specific benefits for mothers-to-be. During pregnancy, most women feel extra strain on their backs. Strengthened back muscles will help you manage the extra weight you will carry, especially by promoting good posture. The elementary and windmill backstroke arm motions can develop your back muscles, helping to alleviate discomfort. In addition, the different leg motions for the backstroke, which can be used interchangeably, are great lower-body toners, especially for the inner and outer thighs, the calves, and buttocks.

This chapter presents the backstroke skills according to arm motions from smaller to larger, in order of increasing difficulty. They include sculling, elementary backstroke, and the windmill backstroke. The flutter kick or breaststroke kick (frog kick) can be used with sculling and elementary backstroke. The windmill backstroke uses the flutter kick.

Sculling

Sculling is a figure-eight motion that is among the most important swimming and balancing skills. Its stability and comfort are especially helpful during pregnancy. The figure-eight motion is used in the basic water safety skill of treading water, as well as in lifesaving and synchronized swimming.

Sculling is efficient because it provides propulsion at every angle; there is continuous positive motion. To achieve this motion, sculling, unlike other strokes, does not have a recovery phase; the figure-eight has no resting motion, and your hand does not leave the water as in the recovery phase of most strokes.

Body Position

Float on your back (supine position) with your legs extended. Your chin should be tipped slightly forward, and your eyes should look down toward your feet. Your general body position will vary according to your stroke and the stage of your pregnancy.

Arm Motion

Sculling uses arm movements similar to those used in treading water. Place your arms at your sides at hip level, parallel to the pool's bottom, with your thumbs up and your palms facing each other. Now make a figure-eight motion (like an infinity sign) with each hand (see Figure 11.1). Turn your thumbs down and press your arms out away from each other until they're about shoulder-width apart; then turn your thumbs up again and press your arms toward each other until your palms are under your hips. Remember to point your fingers upward by flexing your wrists, which will help in propulsion.

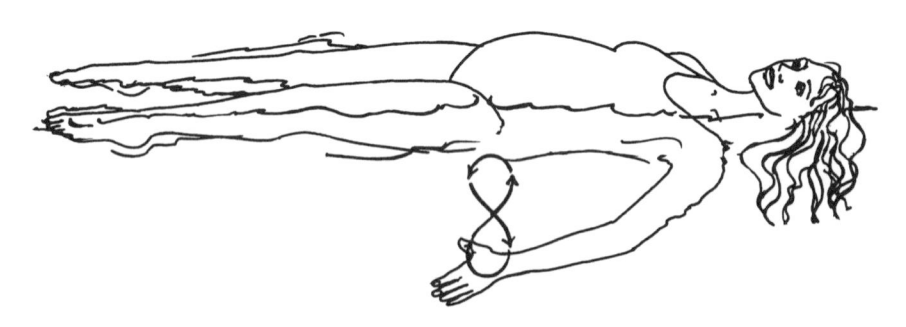

Figure 11.1 The backstroke sculling arm motion.

Leg Motion

Use either an easy flutter kick or a breaststroke kick while sculling.

Breathing

Even though your face is out of the water, you must still pay attention to your breathing. Your breathing should be rhythmic; you should continuously inhale and exhale while on your back.

Stroke Coordination

Your arms and legs should move continuously. However, because the arm motions are small, you don't need to time your arm and leg motions in sculling. Breathe continuously and never hold your breath.

Vertical Treading With Hand Paddles

You may alternate vertical treading with sculling in a back-float position. Treading water is a combination of a figure-eight sculling arm motion and a breaststroke kick in a vertical position (see Figure 11.2). You can use hand paddles for extra upper-body muscle toning. Treading in place is a good exercise if the pool is too crowded for safe and comfortable lap swimming.

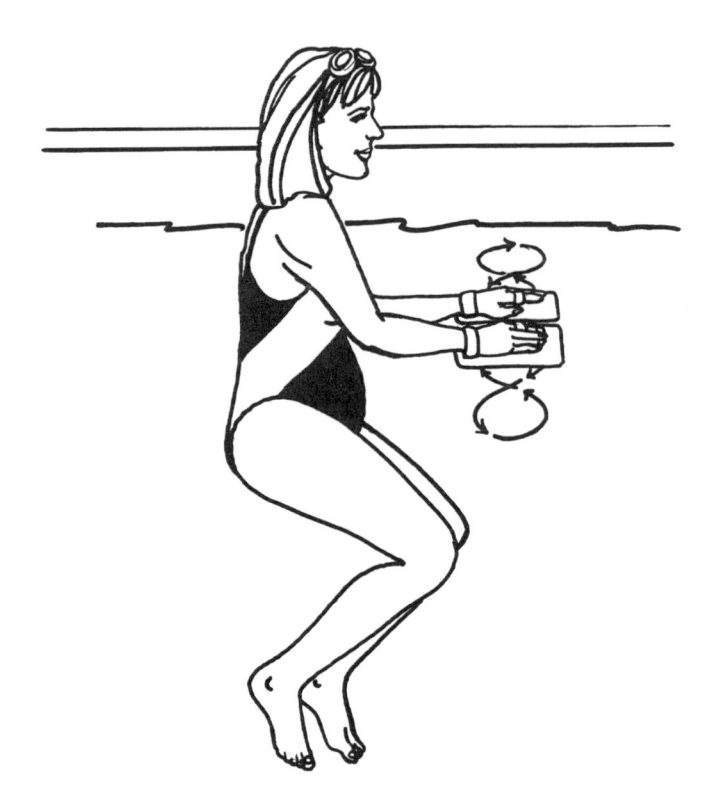

Figure 11.2 Vertical treading with hand paddles.

Elementary Backstroke

In the elementary backstroke, all the arm and leg movements are under the water. The body position is the same as in sculling.

Arm Motion

To begin, your arms should be straight and at your sides. This is the resting or *glide* position (see Figure 11.3). Slide your fingertips along your sides up to your underarms for the *recovery*. Extend your arms outward from the shoulders, beneath the surface of the water, with your palms facing downward in a *V* position for the *catch*. Your hands should be no higher than the top of the head. Pause for a moment before pressing your arms straight downward to your outer thighs for the *pull* (the power part of the stroke). Hold your arms in this glide position momentarily before you begin the cycle again.

Leg Motion

The elementary backstroke usually uses the breaststroke (frog, whip, or modified whip) kick; however you can also use the back flutter kick, if it is more comfortable for you.

Begin the kick on your back with your feet close together near the water's surface. With one movement, bend your knees, drop your heels, and flex your feet toward the bottom of the pool. Next turn your feet outward as you extend your legs to a *V* position. Then bring your legs together with one movement so that your ankles meet. Your legs don't break the surface of the water during the kick.

Breathing

Again, with your face out of the water, no specific breathing pattern is necessary. Breathe fully and continuously, and never hold your breath.

Stroke Coordination

The elementary backstroke begins in a back-float position, with your arms at your sides and your feet together; your arms and legs will move simultaneously. As you draw your arms up along the side of your body, bend your knees and lower your heels. When you extend your arms into a *V* position, your legs will also be in a *V* position. Pull your arms down under the water to your sides as you bring your feet together in this sequence: bend, extend, push arms and legs together, and glide. Rest during the glide and let the momentum of your stroke propel you through the water. Exhale during the power phase (pull) of the stroke, and inhale during the recovery phase.

Windmill Backstroke

In the windmill backstroke you alternately move your arms and use an out-of-the-water arm recovery with a back flutter kick. Again, your body position is the same as in the other two backstrokes.

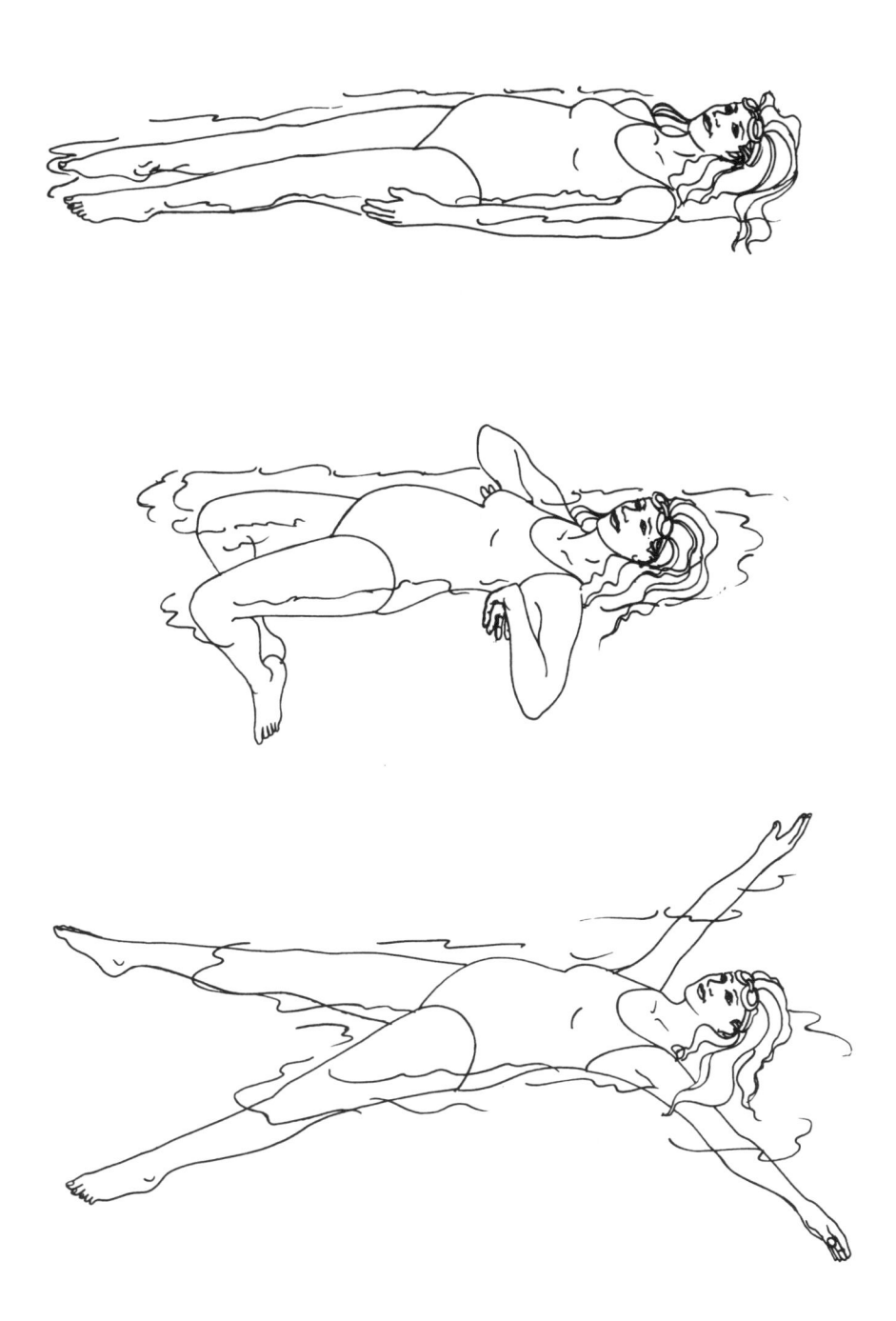

Figure 11.3 The elementary backstroke arm motion.

Arm Motion

In the windmill backstroke, as in the crawl, each arm strokes alternately from the shoulder, with one pulling underwater while the other returns to the starting position.

Beginning from a back-float position, with your arms at your sides, begin the *recovery* by lifting one arm straight up and overhead near the midline of your body (see Figure 11.4). Then bring your hand below the water's surface, with your pinky down, for the *catch*. For the *pull*, bring your arm in back of you in a semicircle. As your thumb touches your outer thigh, rotate your hand so that your little finger starts the *recovery*. While the first arm is in midair recovering, the other arm is pulling. Keep your arms moving continuously and in opposition to each other.

Leg Motion

Use a continuous flutter kick with your windmill backstroke. Bend your knees slightly as you kick your legs alternately toward the surface. Keep your ankles relaxed, and make the water "boil" by just breaking the surface of the water with your feet.

Breathing

There is no specific breathing coordination for this backstroke. As usual, however, breathe fully and continuously.

Stroke Coordination

The coordination of arms, legs, and breathing involves one breath and six kicks per arm cycle. (An arm cycle is one right-arm and left-arm pull.) Inhale and exhale continuously so that you complete a full breath every stroke cycle.

Bent-Arm S-Pull Refinement

For more efficient backstroke propulsion, you can try the S-pull variation by bending your arms as you pull. This is the same principle as the S-shaped pull for the crawl stroke.

In this bent-arm pull, rotate your arms downward from the shoulder (see Figure 11.5 on page 110). Bend your arm at the elbow while under the water at shoulder level; your hand will press more water toward your feet. The extra resistance of the water being pressed toward your feet gives you more propulsion in the forward direction.

Push-Off

The backstroke push-off should be done gently. If you are accustomed to a racing start, wait until your postpartum period is complete before you resume doing it.

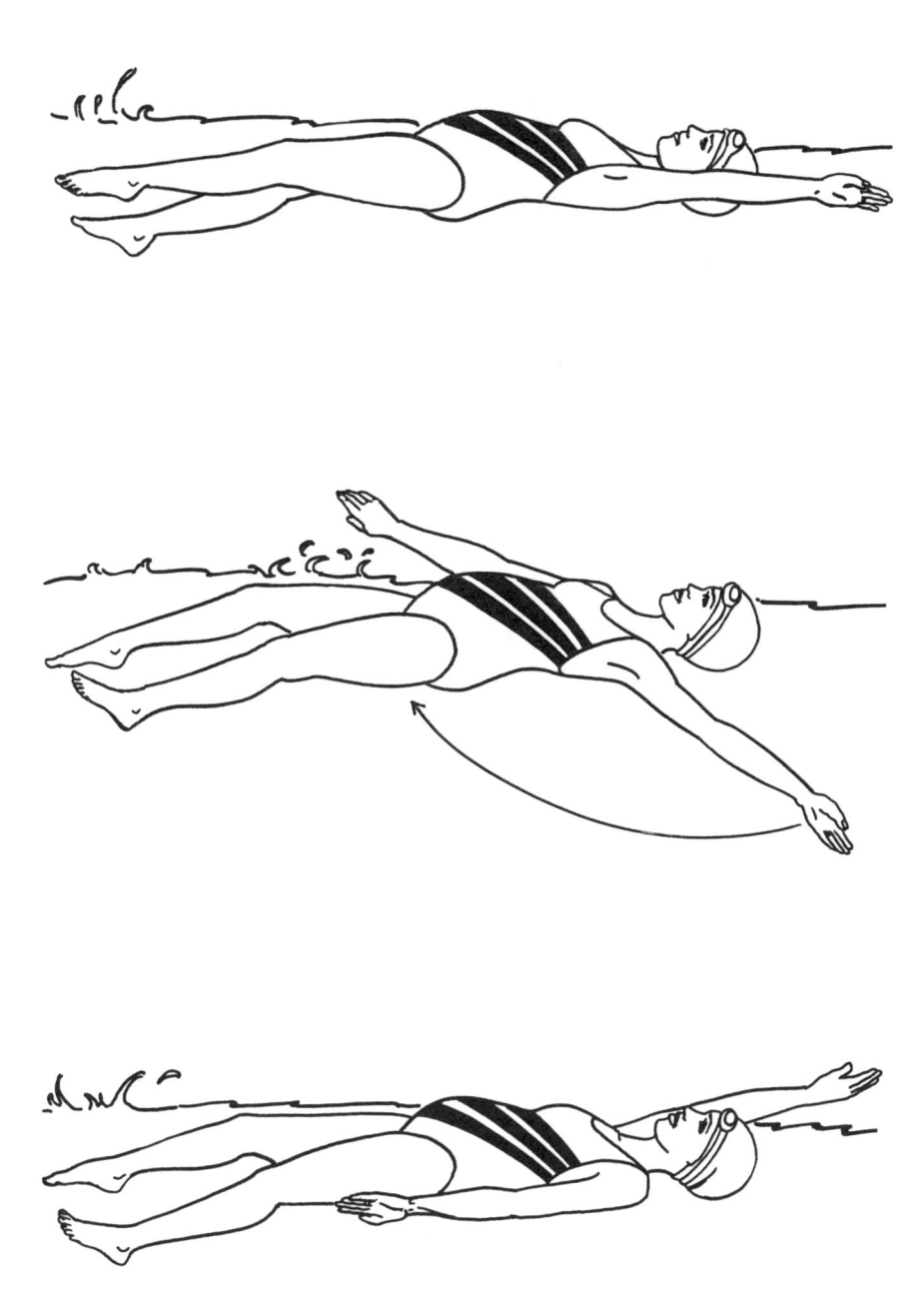

Figure 11.4 The windmill backstroke arm motion.

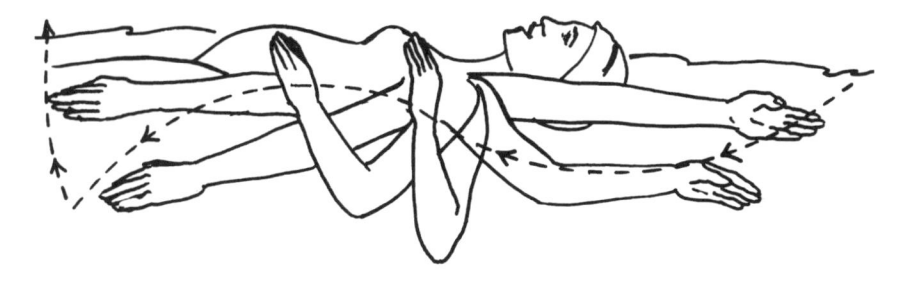

Figure 11.5 The S-pull variation for the windmill backstroke.

To begin your backstroke, face the wall and hold on with both hands with your elbows slightly bent (see Figure 11.6). Place both feet comfortably against the wall below the water's surface. Bring your body into a slightly tucked position by bending your elbows a little more. Gently swing your arms to an over-the-head position. As you extend on your back, try to keep your hips close to the water's surface as you push off with your legs and glide. Before you start swimming, your head should be aligned with your body; your arms should be overhead, covering your ears during the glide, and your body should be streamlined and stretched out.

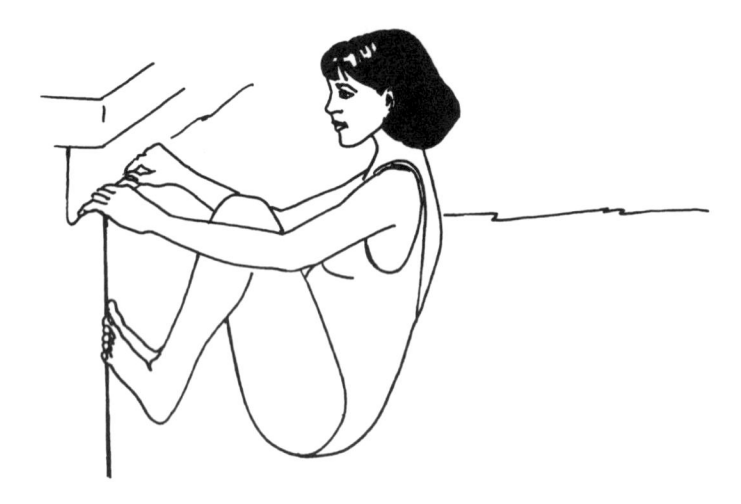

Figure 11.6 The backstroke push-off.

Turn

No matter which backstroke arm motion you use, your turn will be the same. As you reach the wall, extend one hand overhead and grasp the pool's edge (see Figure 11.7). Turn 180° in the direction of the arm that is on the wall, bending and lifting your knees as you turn. Keep your free

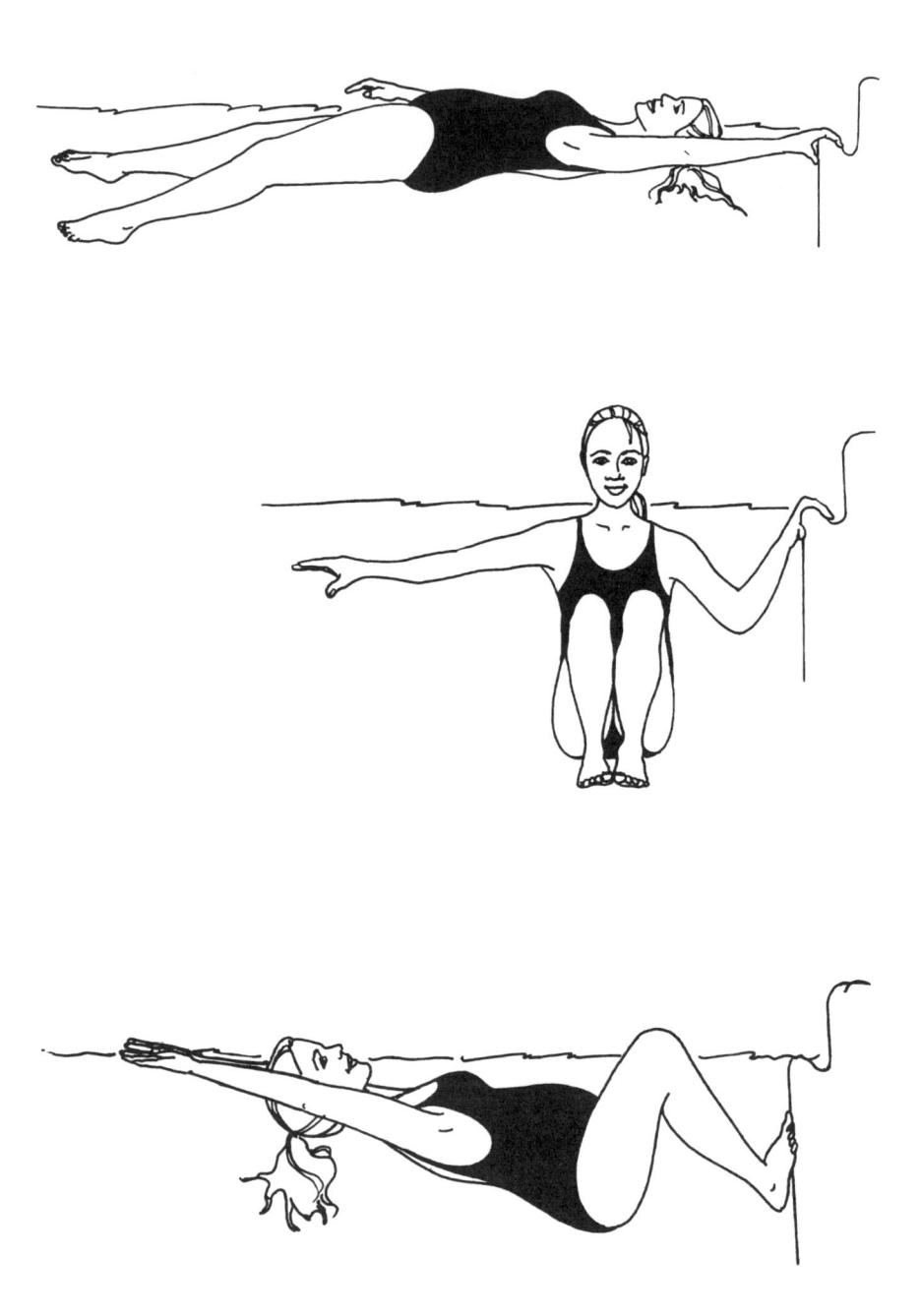

Figure 11.7 The backstroke open turn.

arm extended on the surface of the water. Place your feet comfortably on the wall for your push-off. You should be facing the wall as you push off. As you push off, extend both arms overhead for streamlined body position.

As you approach the wall at the end of the lap, mentally mark a landmark in the pool—such as a ladder, window, flag, or chair—to help you gauge your glide into the wall. Count your strokes from the mark to the wall. Look over your shoulder with the last armstroke as you come to the wall and make contact with your hand. Your ability to judge the distance between your body and the end of the pool will improve with practice.

Backstroke Tips

- Swim the backstroke to give your eyes a rest from wearing goggles.
- Including backstroke in your water fitness program may help keep your lower back comfortable during your pregnancy.
- Experiment with the bent-arm pull (S-pull variation) in the windmill backstroke.
- If you rotate your upper body toward your pulling arm in the windmill backstroke, it will help prevent your hips from swaying. This increases torso toning—another plus for labor and delivery.
- As your pregnancy progresses, you may need to slow down somewhat. Listen to your body and adjust your stroke and stroke coordination as needed.
- As pregnancy progresses, most women swim deeper in the water. Therefore, when you use the flutter kick for the windmill backstroke your feet may no longer break the water's surface. However, you will still get forward movement from your flutter kick.
- During backstroke, be careful of other swimmers. Also be careful about the pool wall—check at periodic intervals to see how far away you are.

48

SCULL AND HUG

Benefits

Strengthens the upper arms and gives practice in the sculling arm motion.

Starting Position

Stand in chest-deep water, feet hip-width apart, with your arms extended in front of you under the water with your palms down.

How to Do It

1. Gently sweep your arms outward and then behind your hips, pressing the water backward.
2. Then reverse the sweep and press water forward with your palms, turning your thumbs up.
3. Move your palms to face and pass each other until your arms hug your body at shoulder level. Breathe normally.

Exercise Tips

- Alternate your arm position at the "hug"—left arm over right, then right over left at the next repetition.
- Be sure not to overstretch, especially when your arms are behind you. (Remember that your ligaments are softer during pregnancy, so you won't necessarily be aware if you have gone too far.)

49

BACK FLUTTER KICK

Benefits

Practices the back flutter kick in a stationary position; tones abdominal and leg muscles.

Starting Position

Place your back against the wall. Hold onto the pool edge, with arms extended to either side.

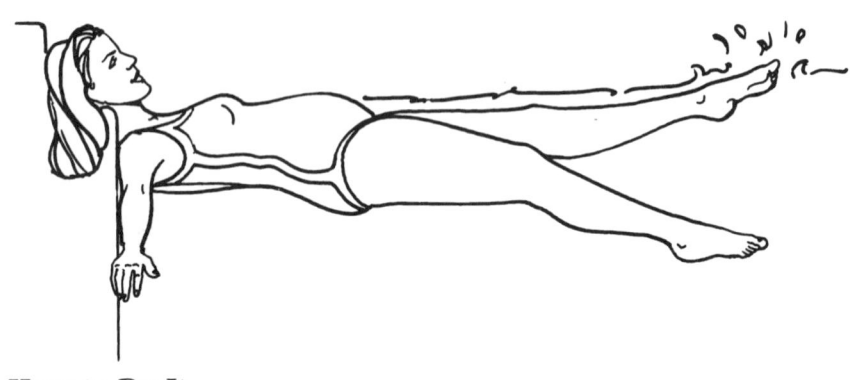

How to Do It

1. Bring your legs up to the surface, adding the back flutter kick. Breathe regularly.
2. Just barely break the water's surface, making the water "boil."

Exercise Tip

- This exercise works best in a pool with the water as high as the deck.

chapter 12

SIDESTROKE

The sidestroke is an excellent stroke that you can use during your entire pregnancy. It is a combination of the breaststroke and the elementary backstroke, with similar leg motions and a long glide underwater. It is a graceful and restful stroke that you will especially enjoy during the later stages of your pregnancy. Another advantage is that your face remains above the water, giving you a full view as you swim and the chance to breathe out of the water.

The Stroke

In the sidestroke, the arms move in opposition: one pulls as the other recovers. The sidestroke has eight variations: two scissors kicks (regular and inverted) and two arm motions (regular and overarm), that can be done on either side for a total of eight variations. You will probably have a favorite combination, but give each of the others a try.

Body Position
Begin the sidestroke with your body floating on either side in a horizontal position. Keep your cheek on the water so that your mouth is out of the water and you are able to breathe continuously. Your body simulates the movement of an accordion: It begins in a streamlined position, contracts to a tuck position, and then returns to a stretched-out position again.

Arm Motion
Your starting position begins at the glide. Extend your lower or bottom arm overhead, in line with your body. Rest your upper or top arm along your upper side with your hand on your thigh (see Figure 12.1).

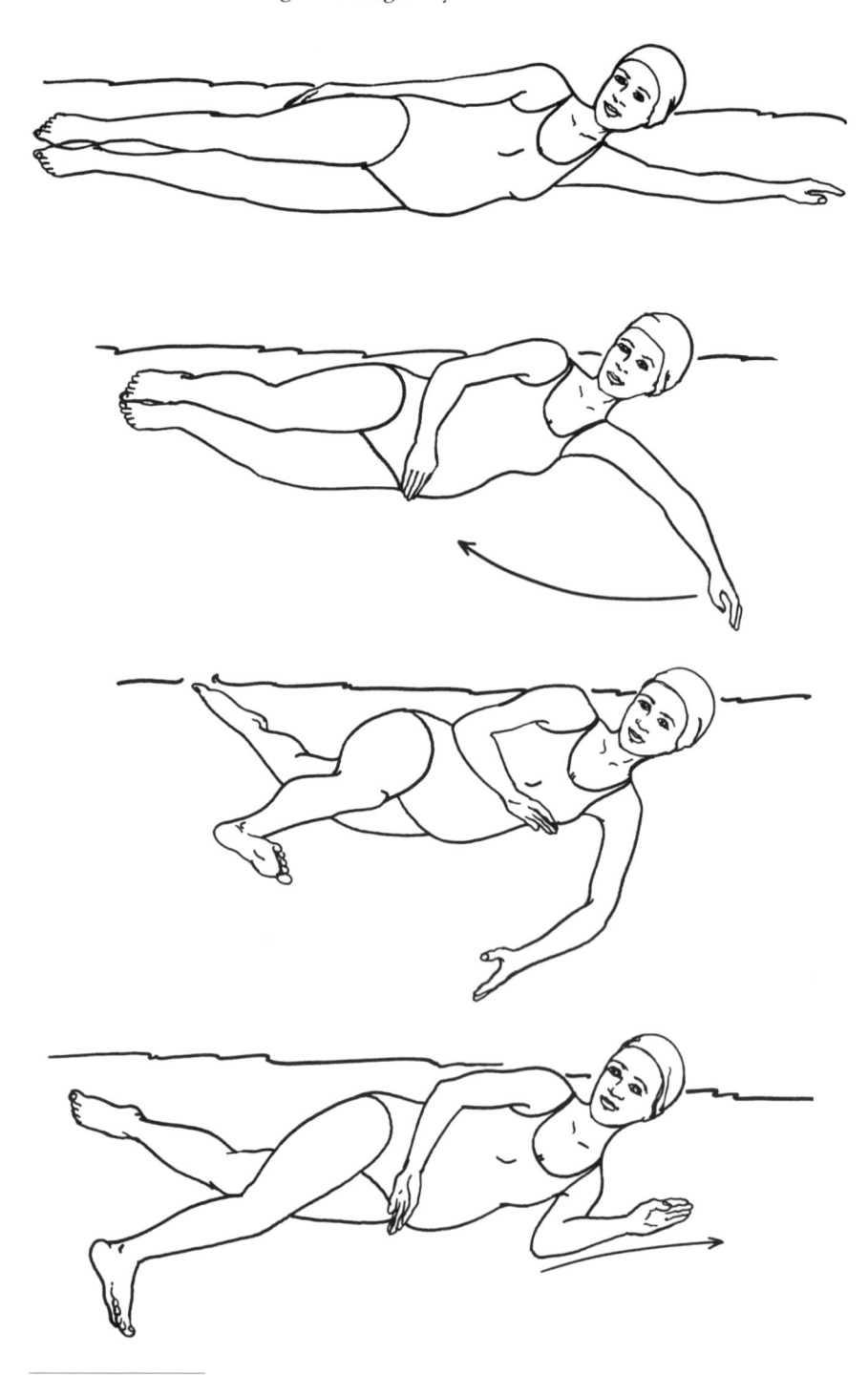

Figure 12.1 The sidestroke arm motion.

As with all other arm strokes, each sidestroke arm motion has a *catch*, a *pull* (power phase), and a *recovery*. Both arms remain underwater throughout the stroke cycle. Remember, as one arm pulls, the other arm recovers—as the top arm (closest to the water's surface) recovers, the bottom or deeper arm pulls, and vice versa.

For the regular sidestroke, begin the *catch* of your lower (bottom) arm by bending your elbow. Then push the water downward toward your feet until your hand is at chest level. To *recover*, bring your elbow close to your side, as in a tuck position. Then extend your arm past your head, back to the starting, or glide, position.

At the same time, your upper (top) arm recovers by sliding the hand toward your chest. The *catch* begins with your palms facing your legs. Push the water toward your feet. When your arm is completely extended, place it at your thigh again and hold it there during the streamlined glide.

If you do the sidestroke with a top-arm recovery, your arm motion will likewise have a *catch*, a *pull*, and a *recovery*. In this variation, the top arm recovers as in the crawl stroke's high-elbow recovery out of the water. The rest of the arm stroke cycle is the same.

Leg Motion

The sidestroke leg motion is called the scissors kick. For conditioning, flexibility, tone, and strength of your inner thigh muscles, the four variations of the scissors kick are great.

In the scissors kick, your legs separate and then come together like a pair of blades. Start in the glide position on your side with your legs extended and your toes pointed. Bring your knees toward your abdomen, approaching a 90° angle between your body and thighs. Your feet should be flexed. Separate your legs, with the top leg staying forward and the bottom leg moving backward to form a *V*. Keep your top foot flexed and point your bottom foot as you extend your legs to a wider *V* position. For propulsion, press your legs together while you're pointing both your feet. This returns you to your streamlined glide position.

For the *inverted scissors kick*, begin as before, but move your bottom leg forward and your top leg backward. Continue with the propulsion phase as in the regular scissors kick.

Breathing

Although your head remains out of the water, keep your breathing rhythmic—inhale as your body tucks and exhale as you glide. You can breathe easily using the sidestroke because your face is out of the water.

Stroke Coordination

From your extended glide position, the first phase of the stroke cycle brings your arms and legs together to a tuck position. During the second phase of the stroke cycle, both the arms and legs extend back to the streamlined position. Inhale as your arms come together in the tuck position. Exhale as you glide. The sidestroke's tuck body position stretches your lower back and can help alleviate lower-back pain.

Push-Off

For the sidestroke push-off, stand perpendicular to the pool wall and hold the wall with your inside hand (the arm closer to the wall). Bend your arm at the elbow (see Figure 12.2). Then extend your other arm forward in the direction you will be swimming. Rest your cheek on the water's surface so that your body will be in the proper alignment, then gently push off the wall and start your sidestroke.

Turns

There are two ways to turn while swimming the sidestroke. The first way is used if you swim on only one side. For this turn, touch the wall with your extended arm (see Figure 12.3). Then tuck your knees slightly toward your chest as you bring the other arm to the wall. Complete the turn by releasing your forward arm from the wall. Finish with your push-off; you will face the opposite side of the pool.

The second way to turn is for the versatile sidestroker who can swim on either side. Begin by touching the wall with the extended arm. As you

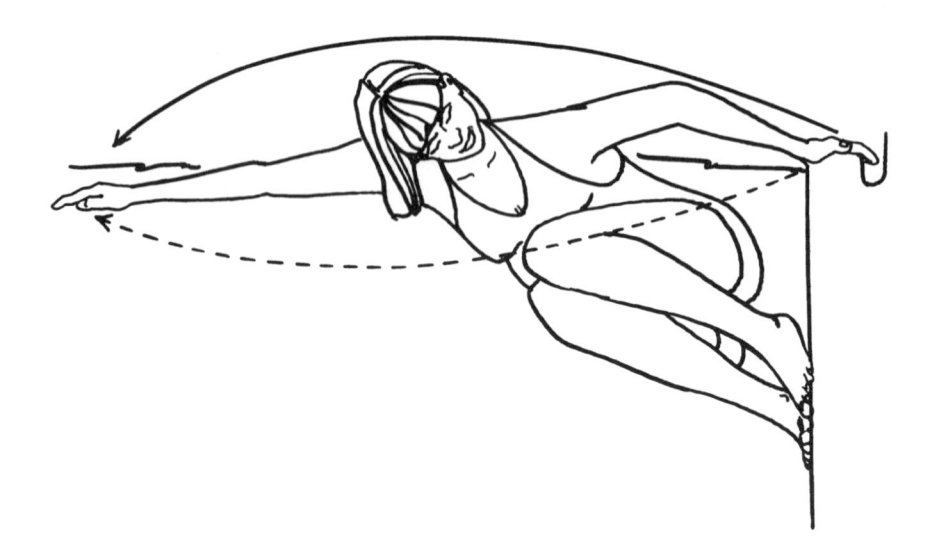

Figure 12.2 The sidestroke push-off.

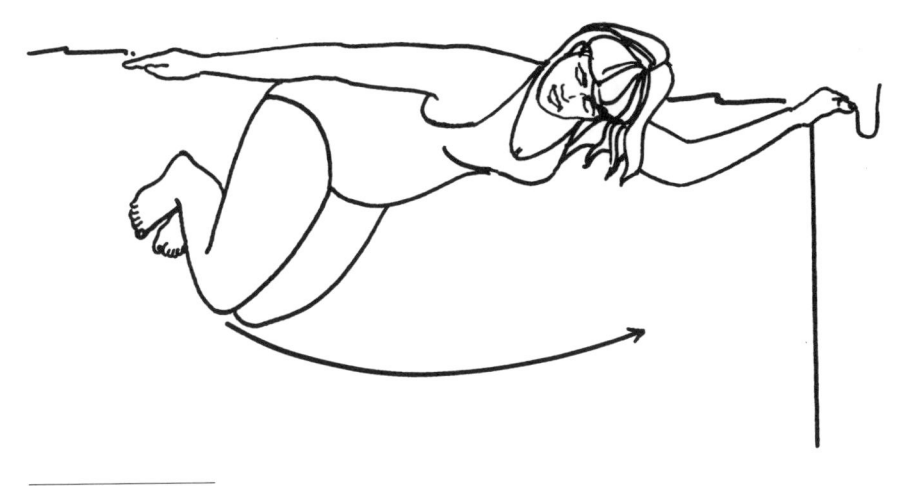

Figure 12.3 The sidestroke turn.

tuck your knees, place your feet on the wall. You will be facing the same direction as before. Complete the turn by using your sidestroke push-off.

Sidestroke Tips

- Because you can look in the direction you are swimming, you do not have to be overly concerned about colliding with other swimmers.
- Try to look slightly ahead so you can keep a better eye on pool traffic. Remember to look, listen, and stay to the right in your lane if you are circling counterclockwise.
- Use the top-arm (high-elbow) recovery variation for extra balance as your pregnancy advances.
- The sidestroke helps stretch, condition, and develop the muscles on your sides and torso.
- The *trudgen* crawl (a crawl arm motion with scissors kick) can be a comfortable stroke during your third trimester. You can use either the regular or inverted scissors kick.

50

UNDER AND OVER

Benefits

Stretches and strengthens arms and shoulders while allowing you to practice the two sidestroke arm motions.

Starting Position

Stand in chest-deep water with feet spaced comfortably apart.

How to Do It

1. Alternately change from the regular arm stroke to the overarm stroke in a pattern such as two overarm and then two regular strokes, and repeat. Breathe fully and continuously.
2. Practice on both sides.

Variation

- Do the exercise in a streamlined glide position on either side to practice.

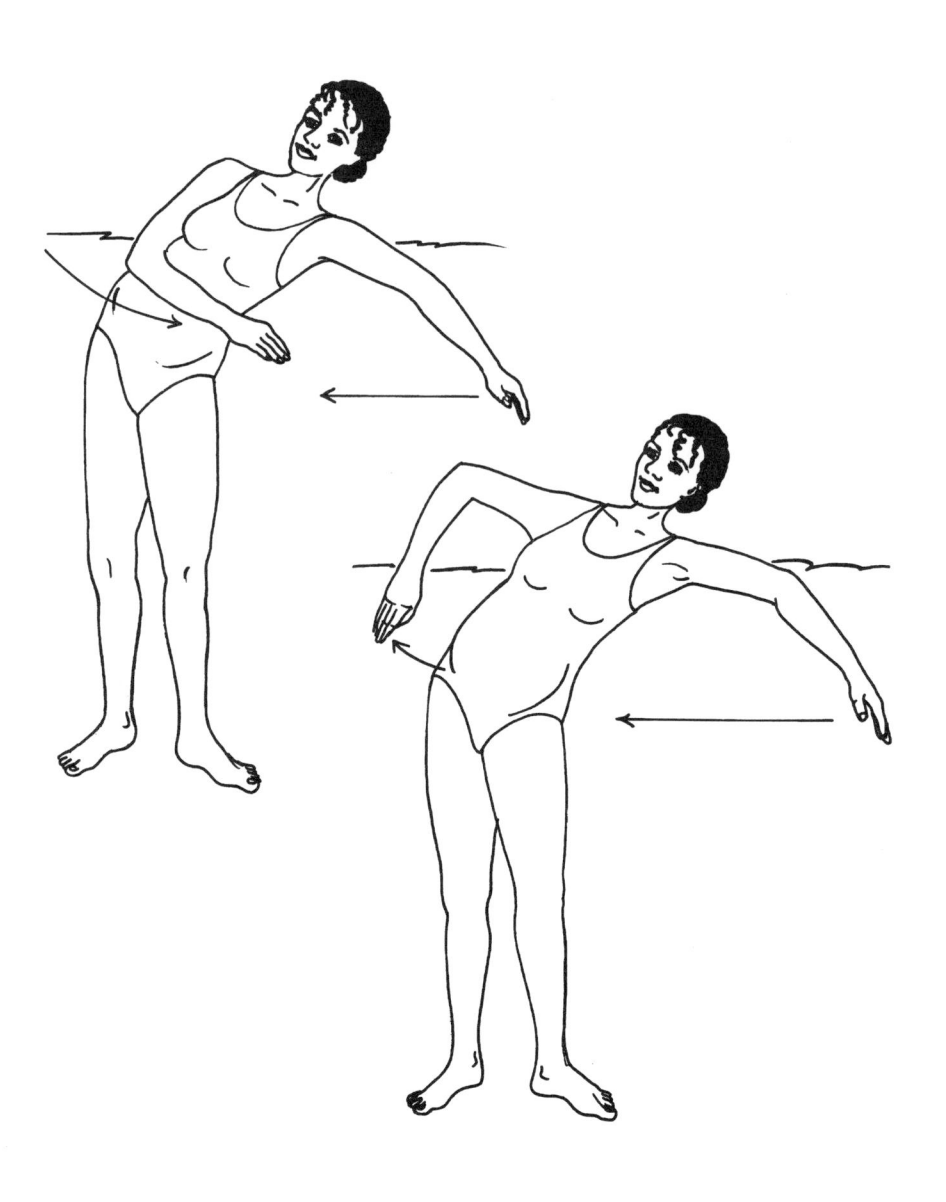

Sidestroke 121

51

Apple Picking

Benefits

Stretches and strengthens arms and shoulders while helping you learn sidestroke arm motion coordination.

Starting Position

Stand in chest-deep water with feet spaced comfortably apart.

How to Do It

1. Extend one arm overhead, reach, and "pick an apple from the tree."
2. Place the "apple" in the other hand at chest level, then throw it downward with that hand (as if into a basket).
3. Reach for another "apple" and repeat. Breathe regularly.
4. Then bring your hands underwater, arms extended sideways. Practice Apple Picking underwater.

Exercise Tip

- Practice on both sides.

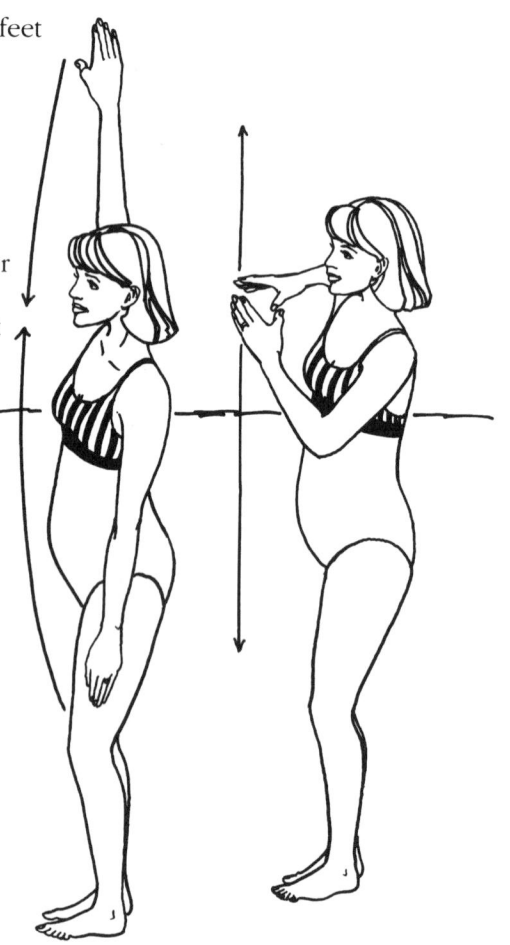

part IV

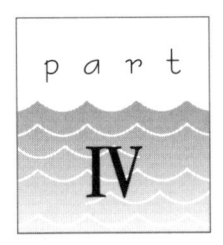

YOUR WATER FITNESS PROGRAM

Part IV details the water exercise and lap swimming programs for each trimester of your pregnancy. Chapter 13 covers the first trimester; chapter 14, the second trimester; and chapter 15, the last trimester. Each chapter describes the body's changes during those months and explains how water fitness can help you. Each chapter also contains month-by-month progressive water exercise workouts designed to take you through your pregnancy, followed by lap swimming workouts. You can use these workouts as they are or mix and match them for your own custom-designed program.

This program begins in the first trimester during the second month of your pregnancy—by that time you will have confirmed your pregnancy and checked with your doctor about exercise. This water fitness program is designed to span the length of your pregnancy. However, your delivery could actually occur anywhere from 2 weeks before your estimated date of confinement (EDC) or due date to 2 weeks after (for a gestation period or term of pregnancy of 38 to 42 weeks). Your pregnancy will actually be more like 10 lunar months than 9 calendar months. Although there is no reason to avoid swimming in your last month, check with your doctor.

The first part of this water fitness program is progressive; sessions gradually increase in content during your first two trimesters. In your third trimester, your workouts will decrease in both time and intensity.

Water exercise workouts are ideal when

- you're not a swimmer yet;

- you can't swim laps because the pool is too small or irregularly shaped;
- the pool is too crowded to swim safely and comfortably;
- you forgot your goggles or you don't want to get your hair or face wet;
- your energy level is low or you don't feel like swimming, but you want to be conscientious about maintaining your conditioning.

You can exercise morning, noon, or night—whenever you prefer. Swim whenever you feel best—if you have morning sickness, swim when you feel better. Don't forget that this program may help you through the uncomfortable parts of your pregnancy.

You may swim one day per week or daily—it depends on you and how you feel. Try to swim every other day, or at least two to three times per week, to achieve maximum benefit. Design your swimming schedule to suit your needs.

According to Jane Hess, DO, family physician and fellow in the sports medicine program at Hennepin County Medical Center in Minneapolis, pregnant women should eat a light meal or a healthful snack about a half hour before exercising, especially during the last trimester. This protects against drastic drops in your blood sugar level. (You may notice that you become uncomfortably hungry after exercising.)

Start your exercise program gradually, especially if you are not accustomed to exercising. You will be more comfortable and derive more benefit if you start out slowly and then expand your program as your muscle tone and aerobic capacity improve.

Generally, pregnant women find that certain swimming strokes are more comfortable than others. Experiment to see which strokes are best for you during the different stages of your pregnancy.

Each water fitness workout has three parts: a warm-up, a main set, and a cool-down. The warm-up takes approximately 5 minutes and prepares your body for exercising. A good warm-up, followed by easy stretches, helps make the main set more comfortable. The main set is the central part of the exercise workout, in which you improve your muscle tone, breathing capacity, and flexibility. It should last from 10 to 20 minutes. Each main swim set has three levels of varying intensity, for women who exercise occasionally, regularly, or frequently. Select the intensity that is appropriate to your fitness level and comfort as highlighted in Table 1. Don't hesitate to switch levels whenever you want to change the intensity of your program. The cool-down helps keep your body loose and limber, and it will bring your body back to a relaxed state after exercising. It should take about 5 minutes.

Table 1 Guide to Swimming Levels

Level	Appropriate for	Frequency of workout	Approximate swim	Warm-up	Main set	Cool-down	Total workout time
1	Occasional exerciser	1 time weekly	25 yards in 1 min	5 min	10 min WETS or laps	5 min	20 min
2	Regular exerciser	2 times weekly	50 yards in 1½ min	5 min	15 min WETS or laps	5 min	25 min
3	Frequent exerciser	3 times weekly or daily	50 yards in 1 min	5 min	20 min WETS or laps	5 min	30 min or more

Most pools are measured in yards or in meters. You can adjust your swim session to accommodate either. The following measurements will help you judge the distance you swim:

- 400 meters = $1/4$ mile (440 yards)
- 800 meters = $1/2$ mile (880 yards)
- In a 20-yard pool
  22 laps = $1/4$ mile
  44 laps = $1/2$ mile
- In a 25-yard pool
  18 laps = $1/4$ mile
  36 laps = $1/2$ mile
- In a 25-meter pool
  16 laps = $1/4$ mile
  32 laps = $1/2$ mile
- In a 50-meter pool
  8 laps = $1/4$ mile
  16 laps = $1/2$ mile

Pools range from classic rectangular, 50-meter Olympic style to an asymmetrical kidney shape. You can use any size or shape pool for your swim sessions although you may have to adjust your exercises slightly to fit the pool.

Keep the following points in mind as you embark on your water exercise program.

- For variety, change strokes or use equipment, such as a kickboard or hand paddles.
- Rest adequately between exercises and swims in your program. Do not push yourself too hard. Your exercise should be mildly challenging but not too taxing. As your pregnancy progresses, give yourself extra rest.
- Vary your resting time between laps according to your comfort, fatigue, and ability level.
- For each trimester use the personal water fitness log in the appendix to record your workouts.
- Enter the pool by sliding in from a sitting position on the wall or use the ladder.
- Keep your doctor fully advised of your exercise program.
- If you experience any discomfort or pain, slow down and take it easy. If the discomfort and pain are more than the "kinks" that result from exercising muscles that aren't used to exercise, or if discomfort continues, stop exercising and check with your doctor.

- Take extra care walking in the pool area and locker room. The floors may be slippery when wet, and pregnancy changes your sense of balance. Wear water shoes to prevent slipping and to keep your feet safe from infection.
- Be meticulous in the care of your feet because you are more susceptible to skin infection during pregnancy.
- If your membranes (bag of waters) rupture in the water, you may feel a gush of warm water as you're swimming. In that case, leave the pool and call your physician immediately!
- *Safety first!* Never overexert yourself and always use caution. Listen at all times to your body—stop swimming if you feel too cold, too hot, or too tired.
- Enjoy yourself!

chapter 13

FIRST-TRIMESTER WORKOUTS

Your first trimester is an exciting time during which you'll be adjusting to the idea of your increasing family size. Your water fitness program helps prepare you physically and emotionally for pregnancy by conditioning your body.

The first-trimester water exercise program starts with the fifth week of pregnancy. By this time you have your doctor's confirmation that you are pregnant and approval to begin this program. However, you may begin this program at any time before or during your pregnancy.

During your first trimester you may experience minor discomforts, such as fatigue, occasional nausea, and frequent urination. Exercising in the water as often as you can may help you feel better and more fit during this time.

You also may feel quite fatigued during your first trimester because of the hormonal changes and other physiological changes your body is undergoing. You'll feel better and keep your spirits up if you swim. Adjust your swim sessions to your own schedule and try to swim when you're not rushed. Even if you feel tired or uncomfortable before you swim, the water and exercise will make you feel better.

Remember, as I have frequently stressed, do not jump or dive into the pool while you're pregnant. Enter the water gently and gracefully, using the ladder or steps. Or sit on the deck with your legs in the water, place your hands on the sides of your hips at the pool edge, press down, and make a quarter turn as you slip into the water.

This chapter includes two sample water exercise workouts and two lap swim workouts for each month in your first trimester. Each sample workout offers three levels of intensity. In addition, you are encouraged to customize a water fitness workout for your own preferences, fitness, and skill level.

Month 2

These beginning water exercise workouts aim to improve your overall fitness level and help tone your muscles. As with all the workouts in this book, these workouts are not "set in stone"; they can provide a guideline or starting point for you to begin your pregnancy water exercise program.

WATER EXERCISE WORKOUT 1

Warm-up (5 minutes)

2	Sit and Kick
4	Water Walk/Jog
12	Breathe and Reach
3	Feet Flex
1	Overhead Stretch

Main set

Level 1 (10 minutes)   1 minute per exercise
                          Rest whenever needed.
Level 2 (15 minutes) $1^1/_2$ minutes per exercise
                          Rest every second exercise.
Level 3 (20 minutes)   2 minutes per exercise
                          Rest every third exercise.

18	Arm Circle
49	Back Flutter Kick
25	Hip Touch
32	Bicycle Pedal
27	Modified Sit-Up
40	Pendulum Body Swing
41	Treading
36	Leg Lift
17	Arm Press
39	Arm and Leg Reach

Cool-down (5 minutes)

13	Breathing With Head Circles
4	Water Walk/Jog
8	Water Kegel
5	Shoulder Shrug
9	Aqua Lunge

WATER EXERCISE WORKOUT 2

Warm-up (5 minutes)

2	Sit and Kick
4	Water Walk/Jog
3	Feet Flex
12	Breathe and Reach
1	Overhead Stretch

Main set

Level 1 (10 minutes) 1 minute per exercise
Rest whenever needed.
Level 2 (15 minutes) $1\frac{1}{2}$ minutes per exercise
Rest every second exercise.
Level 3 (20 minutes) 2 minutes per exercise
Rest every third exercise.

16	Medley of Pulls
31	Flutter Kick
44	Rhythmic Breathing
45	Catch-Up Arm Stroke
47	Frog Kick
20	Hang 10
46	Breaststroke Arm Pull
38	Double Leg Circle
21	Sculling
41	Treading

Cool-down (5 minutes)

- 13 Breathing With Head Circles
- 4 Water Walk/Jog
- 8 Water Kegel
- 5 Shoulder Shrug
- 9 Aqua Lunge

Lap Swim Workout 1

Swim Pointer

- Swim for conditioning (resting as needed).

Reminders

Select the swim level that is right for you. Be sure you have received your doctor's approval before starting this program. Always keep in mind your comfort and safety. Listen to your body!

Warm-up (5 minutes)

- 14 Breathe and Bob
- 44 Rhythmic Breathing
- 5 Shoulder Shrug
- 31 Flutter Kick
- 18 Arm Circle

Main swim

Level 1 (10 minutes)

Swim using the crawl stroke, pausing every lap (e.g., 25 yards) or as needed.

Level 2 (15 minutes)

Swim using the crawl stroke, pausing every two laps (e.g., 50 yards) as needed.

Level 3 (20 minutes)

Swim using the crawl stroke, pausing every four laps (e.g., 100 yards) as needed.

Cool-down (5 minutes)

    45 Catch-Up Arm Stroke (2 minutes)
    20 Hang 10 (1 minute)
    41 Treading (1 minute)
    42 Posture Check (1 minute)

Lap Swim Workout 2

Warm-up (5 minutes)

    14 Breathe and Bob
    44 Rhythmic Breathing
     5 Shoulder Shrug
    31 Flutter Kick

Main swim

Level 1 (10 minutes)

Swim continuously for 5 minutes, using the crawl stroke. Rest only as needed between laps.

    Rest 2 minutes.
    Swim 1 × 50 yards crawl.
    Rest 1 minute.
    Swim 1 × 50 yards crawl.

Level 2 (15 minutes)

Swim continuously for 7 minutes, using the crawl stroke. Rest only as needed between laps.

Rest 2 minutes.
Swim 1 × 50 yards crawl.
Rest 1 minute.
Swim 1 × 50 yards using another stroke of your choice.
Rest 1 minute.
Swim 1 × 50 yards crawl.

Level 3 (20 minutes)

Swim continuously for 10 minutes, using the crawl stroke. Rest only as needed between laps.

Rest 3 minutes.
Swim 1 × 50 yards using another stroke of your choice.
Rest 1 minute.
Swim 1 × 50 yards crawl.
Rest 1 minute.
Swim 1 × 50 yards using another stroke of your choice.
Rest 1 minute.
Swim 1 × 50 yards crawl.

Cool-down (5 minutes)

45 Catch-Up Arm Stroke (2 minutes)
20 Hang 10 (1 minute)
41 Treading (1 minute)
42 Posture Check (1 minute)

Month 3

The third month of pregnancy is a good time to start strengthening your back and abdominal muscles because you'll soon need them to support your growing abdomen.

The first of these two workouts is designed with your busy schedule in mind—most of the exercises keep your hair and face out of the water. Sometimes that convenience may make the difference between being able to take time out for your workout and not being able to fit it in.

WATER EXERCISE WORKOUT | 3 |

Warm-up (5 minutes)

2	Sit and Kick
4	Water Walk/Jog
6	Stand Tall
14	Breathe and Bob
1	Overhead Stretch

Main set

Level 1 (10 minutes)   1 minute per exercise
Rest whenever needed.

Level 2 (15 minutes) $1^1/_2$ minutes per exercise
Rest every second exercise.

Level 3 (20 minutes)   2 minutes per exercise
Rest every third exercise.

22	Wall Push-Up
23	Kickboard Press
24	Circle Spray
37	Leg Swirl
29	Wall Knee Lift
28	Swing and Sway
19	Sport Swing
21	Sculling (stand in chest-deep water to keep hair dry)
33	Leg Scissors
42	Posture Check

Cool-down (5 minutes)

5	Shoulder Shrug
8	Water Kegel
4	Water Walk/Jog
7	Pelvic Tilt
12	Breathe and Reach

WATER EXERCISE WORKOUT 4

Warm-up (5 minutes)

2	Sit and Kick
4	Water Walk/Jog
6	Stand Tall
14	Breathe and Bob
1	Overhead Stretch

Main set

Level 1 (10 minutes)   1 minute per exercise
Rest whenever needed.

Level 2 (15 minutes) $1\frac{1}{2}$ minutes per exercise
Rest every second exercise.

Level 3 (20 minutes)   2 minutes per exercise
Rest every third exercise.

17	Arm Press
27	Modified Sit-Up
34	Calf Stretch
38	Double Leg Circle
41	Treading
40	Pendulum Body Swing
20	Hang 10
26	Back Extension
43	Deep-Water Jog
24	Circle Spray

Cool-down (5 minutes)

5	Shoulder Shrug
8	Water Kegel
4	Water Walk/Jog
7	Pelvic Tilt
12	Breathe and Reach

Lap Swim Workout 3

Swim Pointers

- *Stroke-count* means counting the number of strokes per lap. The lower the count, the more efficient your stroke becomes. Count your strokes as your fingertips enter the water (for the catch of each stroke).
- The notation "4 × 25 yards" is used to indicate four repetitions of a 25-yard swim or four laps around a 25-yard pool. Likewise "4 × 50 yards" indicates four repetitions of a 50-yard swim, the equivalent of eight laps around a 25-yard pool.

Reminder

Stretch out and get the most glide from each arm motion.

Warm-up (5 minutes)

14	Breathe and Bob
21	Sculling (2 minutes)
47	Frog Kick
41	Treading

Main swim

Level 1 (10 minutes)

Swim continuously for 5 minutes, varying your strokes.
    Rest for 2 minutes.
    Swim 4 × 25 yards. Count the number of strokes per lap and try to keep that number constant for each lap.

Level 2 (15 minutes)

Swim continuously for 10 minutes, varying your strokes.
    Rest for 2 minutes.
    Swim 4 × 25 yards. Count the number of strokes per lap and try to keep that number constant for each lap.

Level 3 (20 minutes)

Swim continuously for 15 minutes, varying your strokes.
  Rest for 2 minutes.
  Swim 4 × 25 yards. Count the number of strokes per lap and try to keep that number constant for each lap.

Cool-down (5 minutes)

Choose five cool-down exercises.

LAP SWIM WORKOUT 4

Swim Pointers

- "3 × 50 yards on 2 minutes" indicates a method called *interval training*, which is often used by fitness and competitive swimmers in practice. You swim 50 yards three times with the swims beginning 2 minutes apart, using the pace or wall clock or seconds on your wristwatch. The second 50 yards begins exactly 2 minutes after the first, and the third 50 yards begins exactly 2 minutes after the second, and so on. In interval training, the amount of rest you have after each swim is determined by how fast you have been going. It can be used with any variety of strokes, distances, or time intervals.

Warm-up (5 minutes)

14	Breathe and Bob
21	Sculling (2 minutes)
47	Frog Kick
41	Treading

Main swim

Level 1 (10 minutes)

Swim continuously for 2 minutes, using the crawl stroke. Rest between laps only as needed.

> Rest 1 minute.
> Swim 2 × 25 yards, using the breaststroke on 1 minute.
> Rest 1 minute.
> Swim 4 × 25 yards, using the crawl stroke on 1 minute.

Level 2 (15 minutes)

Swim continuously for 4 minutes, using the crawl stroke. Rest between laps only as needed.

> Rest 2 minutes.
> Swim 2 × 25 yards, using the breaststroke on 1 minute.
> Rest 1 minute.
> Swim 2 × 25 yards, using the crawl stroke on 1 minute.
> Rest 2 minutes.
> Swim 2 minutes continuously, using the stroke of your choice.

Level 3 (20 minutes)

Swim continuously for 10 minutes, using the crawl stroke. Rest between laps only as needed.

> Rest 2 minutes.
> Swim 2 × 25 yards, using the breaststroke on 1 minute.
> Rest 1 minute.
> Swim 2 × 25 yards, using the crawl stroke on 1 minute.
> Rest 1 minute.
> Swim 2 minutes continuously using the stroke of your choice.

Cool-down (5 minutes)

Choose five cool-down exercises.

chapter 14

SECOND-TRIMESTER WORKOUTS

During the second trimester your body probably will have adjusted to the changes of the first trimester, and swimming will be easier.

This chapter includes two sample water exercise workouts and two lap swim workouts for each month in your second trimester. Each sample workout offers three levels of intensity. In addition, you are encouraged to customize a water fitness workout for your own preferences, fitness, and skill level.

The highlights of the swim and water fitness workout for the second trimester include an introduction to new water exercises; a review of swimming strokes, including breaststroke, sidestroke, and backstroke variations; an introduction to a medley of strokes; lap counts for distance swims; and water exercise.

Month 4

The fourth month of pregnancy is often the easiest—many women find they are most energetic during the second trimester. Your body has adjusted to pregnancy, but you are not yet carrying too much added weight.

This is an excellent time for a nonswimmer to attain a new level of comfort in the water, a new swimmer to practice stroke skills, and an experienced swimmer to refine swim technique.

WATER EXERCISE WORKOUT 5

Warm-up (5 minutes)

- 2   Sit and Kick
- 3   Feet Flex
- 4   Water Walk/Jog
- 14   Breathe and Bob
- 8   Water Kegel

Main set

Level 1 (10 minutes)   1 minute per exercise
Rest whenever needed.

Level 2 (15 minutes) $1^1/_2$ minutes per exercise
Rest every second exercise.

Level 3 (20 minutes)   2 minutes per exercise
Rest every third exercise.

- 16   Medley of Pulls
- 20   Hang 10
- 21   Sculling
- 31   Flutter Kick
- 26   Back Extension
- 32   Bicycle Pedal
- 38   Double Leg Circle
- 40   Pendulum Body Swing
- 41   Treading
- 34   Calf Stretch

Cool-down (5 minutes)

- 7   Pelvic Tilt
- 9   Aqua Lunge
- 13   Breathing With Head Circles
- 8   Water Kegel
- 1   Overhead Stretch

WATER EXERCISE WORKOUT | 6 |

Warm-up (5 minutes)

2	Sit and Kick
3	Feet Flex
4	Water Walk/Jog
14	Breathe and Bob
8	Water Kegel

Main set

Level 1 (10 minutes)   1 minute per exercise
Rest whenever needed.

Level 2 (15 minutes) $1^1/_2$ minutes per exercise
Rest every second exercise.

Level 3 (20 minutes)   2 minutes per exercise
Rest every third exercise.

23	Kickboard Press
25	Hip Touch
45	Catch-Up Arm Stroke
33	Leg Scissors
42	Posture Check
43	Deep-Water Jog
36	Leg Lift
18	Arm Circle
39	Arm and Leg Reach
50	Under and Over

Cool-down (5 minutes)

7	Pelvic Tilt
9	Aqua Lunge
13	Breathing With Head Circles
8	Water Kegel
1	Overhead Stretch

Lap Swim Workout 5

Swim Pointer

- Focus on the breaststroke.

Reminders

Practice the arm and leg motion. Rest between laps as needed. Use *pyramid swims*—increasing and then decreasing your lap distance—to build up your endurance.

Warm-up (5 minutes)

47	Frog Kick
8	Water Kegel
7	Pelvic Tilt
46	Breaststroke Arm Pull
38	Double Leg Circle

Main swim

Level 1 (10 minutes)

Include a cleansing breath after each swim. Swim the following distances:

- 1 × 25 yards
- 1 × 50 yards
- 1 × 100 yards
- 1 × 50 yards
- 1 × 25 yards

Level 2 (15 minutes)

Include a cleansing breath after each swim. Swim the following distances:

- 1 × 50 yards
- 1 × 75 yards
- 1 × 100 yards
- 1 × 75 yards
- 1 × 50 yards

Level 3 (30 minutes)

Include a cleansing breath after each swim. Swim the following distances:

    1 × 25 yards
    1 × 75 yards
    1 × 100 yards
    1 × 200 yards
    1 × 100 yards
    1 × 75 yards
    1 × 25 yards

Cool-down (5 minutes)

Choose five cool-down exercises.

LAP SWIM WORKOUT 6

Warm-up (5 minutes)

47	Frog Kick
8	Water Kegel
7	Pelvic Tilt
46	Breaststroke Arm Pull
38	Double Leg Circle

Main swim

Level 1 (10 minutes)

Swim continuously for 5 minutes using a stroke of your choice. Rest as needed.
Swim 4 × 25 yards using the breaststroke or sidestroke.

Level 2 (15 minutes)

Swim continuously for 8 minutes using the stroke of your choice.
    Rest as needed.
    Swim 4 × 25 yards using the breaststroke or sidestroke.
    Rest 1 minute.
    Swim 50 yards using the crawl stroke.

Level 3 (20 minutes)

Swim continuously for 10 minutes using the stroke of your choice.
    Rest as needed.
    Swim 3 × 50 yards using the breaststroke or sidestroke.
    Rest 2 minutes.
    Swim 50 yards using the crawl stroke.

Cool-down (5 minutes)

    Choose five cool-down exercises.

Month 5

As your pregnancy progresses, you'll be interested in strengthening and toning your abdominal muscles, as well as staying limber and active. These workouts give attention to your middle body and special attention to your posture.

WATER EXERCISE WORKOUT 7

Warm-up (5 minutes)

2	Sit and Kick
14	Breathe and Bob
6	Stand Tall
20	Hang 10
18	Arm Circle

Main set

Level 1 (10 minutes) 1 minute per exercise
Rest whenever needed.
Level 2 (15 minutes) $1^1/_2$ minutes per exercise
Rest every second exercise.
Level 3 (20 minutes) 2 minutes per exercise
Rest every third exercise.

16	Medley of Pulls
24	Circle Spray
27	Modified Sit-Up
49	Back Flutter Kick
41	Treading
32	Bicycle Pedal
26	Back Extension
36	Leg Lift
40	Pendulum Body Swing
43	Deep-Water Jog (optional—with or without a flotation device)

Cool-down (5 minutes)

8	Water Kegel
39	Arm and Leg Reach
5	Shoulder Shrug
11	Cleansing Breath
25	Hip Touch

WATER EXERCISE WORKOUT 8

Warm-up (5 minutes)

2	Sit and Kick
14	Breathe and Bob
6	Stand Tall
20	Hang 10
18	Arm Circle

Main set

Level 1 (10 minutes)	1 minute per exercise Rest whenever needed.
Level 2 (15 minutes)	1½ minutes per exercise Rest every second exercise.
Level 3 (20 minutes)	2 minutes per exercise Rest every third exercise.

- 28 Swing and Sway
- 37 Leg Swirl
- 44 Rhythmic Breathing
- 23 Kickboard Press
- 19 Sport Swing
- 31 Flutter Kick
- 41 Treading
- 42 Posture Check
- 26 Back Extension
- 22 Wall Push-Up

Cool-down (5 minutes)

- 8   Water Kegel
- 39 Arm and Leg Reach
- 5   Shoulder Shrug
- 11 Cleansing Breath
- 25 Hip Touch

Lap Swim Workout 7

Swim Pointers

- Practice laps while sculling on your back.
- Learn or review the elementary backstroke.

Reminders

Sculling is a figure-eight motion. In the elementary backstroke, both arms and legs move simultaneously. Rest between laps as needed.

Warm-up (5 minutes)

21 Sculling
14 Breathe and Bob
11 Cleansing Breath
47 Frog Kick
41 Treading

Main swim

Level 1 (10 minutes)

Scull 1 × 25 yards.
Take one cleansing breath.
Swim 1 × 50 yards of elementary backstroke.
Take one cleansing breath.
Swim continuously for 3 minutes.
Scull 1 × 25 yards.
Take one cleansing breath.
Swim 1 × 50 yards of elementary backstroke.

Level 2 (15 minutes)

Scull 1 × 25 yards.
Take two cleansing breaths.
Swim 1 × 75 yards of elementary backstroke.
Take two cleansing breaths.
Scull 1 × 25 yards.
Take two cleansing breaths.
Swim 1 × 75 yards of elementary backstroke.

Level 3 (20 minutes)

Scull 1 × 25 yards using your arms only.
Take two cleansing breaths.
Swim 1 × 100 yards of elementary backstroke.
Take two cleansing breaths.
Scull 1 × 25 yards.
Take two cleansing breaths.
Swim 1 × 100 yards of elementary backstroke.

Cool-down (5 minutes)

41	Treading
14	Breathe and Bob
11	Cleansing Breath
33	Leg Scissors
8	Water Kegel

LAP SWIM WORKOUT 8

Warm-up (5 minutes)

21	Sculling
14	Breathe and Bob
11	Cleansing Breath
47	Frog Kick
41	Treading

Main swim

Level 1 (10 minutes)

Using the crawl stroke, swim 4 × 25 yards, beginning a lap every 1 minute and 15 seconds.
Rest as needed.
Swim continuously for 5 minutes, varying your strokes.

Level 2 (15 minutes)

Using the crawl stroke, swim 4 × 25 yards, beginning a lap every 45 seconds.
Rest as needed.
Swim continuously for 5 minutes using the stroke of your choice.
Using the stroke of your choice, swim 4 × 25 yards, beginning a lap every 1 minute and 15 seconds.

Level 3 (20 minutes)

Using the crawl stroke, swim 4 × 50 yards, beginning a lap every 1 minute and 30 seconds.
Rest as needed.
Swim continuously for 5 minutes using the stroke of your choice.
Rest 1 minute.
Using the backstroke or breaststroke, swim 6 × 25 yards, beginning a lap every 45 seconds.

Cool-down (5 minutes)

41	Treading
14	Breathe and Bob
11	Cleansing Breath
33	Leg Scissors
8	Water Kegel

Month 6

These workouts are designed to help prepare you to be *big*. Even if you have only recently begun to "show," this isn't too early to strengthen your back muscles—they will be responsible for offsetting the weight of your growing abdomen. These exercises will help you minimize or avoid the lower-back pain experienced all too frequently during the second half of pregnancy. You may also begin researching prepared childbirth programs available in your area.

For most pregnant women, their sixth month is their most energetic—they feel great and have the exhilaration of looking forward to their new babies.

WATER EXERCISE WORKOUT 9

Warm-up (5 minutes)

14	Breathe and Bob
4	Water Walk/Jog
20	Hang 10
3	Feet Flex
8	Water Kegel

Main set

Level 1 (10 minutes)   1 minute per exercise
                         Rest whenever needed.
Level 2 (15 minutes)   1½ minutes per exercise
                         Rest every second exercise.
Level 3 (20 minutes)   2 minutes per exercise
                         Rest every third exercise.

- 40 Pendulum Body Swing
- 38 Double Leg Circle
- 27 Modified Sit-Up
- 25 Hip Touch
- 32 Bicycle Pedal
- 23 Kickboard Press
- 29 Wall Knee Lift
- 31 Flutter Kick
- 41 Treading
- 30 Back Massage

Cool-down (5 minutes)

- 7   Pelvic Tilt
- 34 Calf Stretch
- 5   Shoulder Shrug
- 9   Aqua Lunge
- 1   Overhead Stretch

WATER EXERCISE WORKOUT 10

Warm-up (5 minutes)

- 14 Breathe and Bob
- 4   Water Walk/Jog
- 20 Hang 10
- 3   Feet Flex
- 8   Water Kegel

Main set

Level 1 (10 minutes) 1 minute per exercise
Rest whenever needed.

Level 2 (15 minutes) 1½ minutes per exercise
Rest every second exercise.

Level 3 (20 minutes) 2 minutes per exercise
Rest every third exercise.

- 24 Circle Spray
- 19 Sport Swing
- 35 Wall Walk
- 43 Deep-Water Jog
- 36 Leg Lift
- 42 Posture Check
- 17 Arm Press
- 26 Back Extension
- 22 Wall Push-Up
- 34 Calf Stretch

Cool-down (5 minutes)

- 13 Breathing With Head Circles
- 7 Pelvic Tilt
- 5 Shoulder Shrug
- 9 Aqua Lunge
- 1 Overhead Stretch

LAP SWIM WORKOUT 9

Swim Pointer

- Increase your conditioning by varying your pace between easy and energetic.
- In this workout, you can combine two strokes, one at an easy pace and another at a moderate pace.

Reminders

Practice a newer stroke at an easy pace; swim a familiar stroke, such as the crawl, at a moderate pace.

Warm-up (5 minutes)

- 49 Back Flutter Kick
- 31 Flutter Kick
- 51 Apple Picking
- 33 Leg Scissors
- 36 Leg Lift

Main swim

Level 1 (10 minutes)

Alternate 25- and 50-yard swims at an easy and moderate pace:

Swim 2 × 25 yards.
Rest for 30 seconds.
Swim 2 × 50 yards.
Rest for 30 seconds.
Swim 2 × 25 yards.

Level 2 (15 minutes)

Alternate 25-, 50-, and 75-yard swims (easy and moderate pace):

Swim 2 × 25 yards.
Rest.
Swim 2 × 50 yards.
Rest.
Swim 2 × 75 yards.
Rest.
Swim 2 × 50 yards.
Rest.
Swim 2 × 25 yards.

Level 3 (20 minutes)

Alternate 50-, 75-, and 100-yard swims (easy and moderate pace):

    Swim 2 × 50 yards.
    Rest.
    Swim 2 × 75 yards.
    Rest.
    Swim 2 × 100 yards.
    Rest.
    Swim 2 × 75 yards.
    Rest.
    Swim 2 × 50 yards.

Cool-down (5 minutes)

28	Swing and Sway
14	Breathe and Bob
18	Arm Circle
8	Water Kegel
41	Treading (deep water optional)

Lap Swim Workout 10

Warm-up (5 minutes)

49	Back Flutter Kick
31	Flutter Kick
51	Apple Picking
33	Leg Scissors
36	Leg Lift

Main swim

Level 1 (10 minutes)

Swim continuously for 5 minutes using the stroke of your choice. Rest as needed. Swim 4 × 25 yards using various strokes. Rest after each lap as needed.

    1 × 25 yards backstroke
    1 × 25 yards breaststroke
    1 × 25 yards sidestroke
    1 × 25 yards crawl stroke

Level 2 (15 minutes)

Swim continuously for 8 minutes using the stroke of your choice. Rest as needed. Swim 4 × 50 yards using various strokes. Rest after 50 yards as needed.

    1 × 50 yards backstroke
    1 × 50 yards breaststroke
    1 × 50 yards sidestroke
    1 × 50 yards crawl stroke

Level 3 (20 minutes)

Swim continuously for 10 minutes using the stroke of your choice. Rest as needed. Swim 4 × 50 yards using various strokes. Rest after 50 yards as needed.

    1 × 50 yards backstroke
    1 × 50 yards breaststroke
    1 × 50 yards sidestroke
    1 × 50 yards crawl stroke
Rest as needed.
Swim 1 × 100 yards using the crawl stroke.
Swim 1 × 50 yards using the stroke of your choice.

Cool-down (5 minutes)

28	Swing and Sway
14	Breathe and Bob
18	Arm Circle
8	Water Kegel
41	Treading (deep water optional)

chapter 15

THIRD-TRIMESTER WORKOUTS

Although you will be larger during the third trimester, you will still be able to swim and exercise. Your water fitness program will help maintain your fitness, strength, and flexibility; and it will be related to the exercises taught in many prepared childbirth programs. You'll probably ease up, so that your workouts will be less demanding than they were during your first and second trimesters. The third trimester program ends at your 36th week. If you want to continue exercising past the 36th week, check with your doctor and keep him or her informed of your progress.

Breathing exercises are especially important during your third trimester. Concentrate on full inhalation and exhalation, and practice breathing patterns combined with effleurage.

During the third trimester, you may experience the return of some discomforts of the first trimester. As the baby drops into the pelvis, you may experience increased frequency of urination, caused by pressure on the bladder. You also may become fatigued more easily because of your extra girth and weight. Take one day at a time during your third trimester, and adjust each water exercise or swim session to your comfort. Avoid any movement or strokes that feel uncomfortable and schedule extra time to relax after your swim. It is recommended that you have a light snack about an hour before your swim to avoid becoming overly hungry.

This chapter includes two sample water exercise workouts and two lap swim workouts for each month in your third trimester. Each sample workout offers three levels of intensity. In addition, you are encouraged to customize a water fitness workout for your own preferences, fitness, and skill level (see the appendix).

The third-trimester water fitness program highlights these elements: cleansing breath, introduction to prepared childbirth breathing exercises used during labor and delivery, increased warm-up and cool-down times, sidestroke variations, and floating and relaxing.

Month 7

The workouts for the third trimester are designed to exercise your muscles to minimize the discomforts of the last trimester and to stretch and strengthen them for the birth. If you are attending a prepared childbirth class, you are probably being introduced to similar exercises on land.

By now you are no doubt appreciating the buoyancy of the water that helps alleviate the heavy feeling of your pregnancy. If you are carrying during warm weather, the pool probably looks good and feels great, too. Keep up the good work!

WATER EXERCISE WORKOUT 11

Warm-up (5 minutes)

4	Water Walk/Jog
2	Sit and Kick
13	Breathing With Head Circles
11	Cleansing Breath
1	Overhead Stretch

Main set

Level 1 (10 minutes)	1 minute per exercise Rest whenever needed.
Level 2 (15 minutes)	$1\frac{1}{2}$ minutes per exercise Rest every second exercise.
Level 3 (20 minutes)	2 minutes per exercise Rest every third exercise.

Safety tip: During the third trimester you may begin to need more rest periods. Add them whenever needed; use these levels as a guide only.

- 26 Back Extension (if you have a back concern, substitute another exercise)
- 17 Arm Press
- 20 Hang 10
- 25 Hip Touch
- 21 Sculling
- 28 Swing and Sway
- 41 Treading
- 37 Leg Swirl
- 35 Wall Walk
- 43 Deep-Water Jog (optional—in deep water, with or without flotation)

Cool-down (5 minutes)

- 6 Stand Tall
- 8 Water Kegel
- 5 Shoulder Shrug
- 9 Aqua Lunge
- 10 Effleurage

WATER EXERCISE WORKOUT | 12 |

Warm-up (5 minutes)

4	Water Walk/Jog
2	Sit and Kick
13	Breathing With Head Circles
11	Cleansing Breath
1	Overhead Stretch

Main set

Level 1 (10 minutes)   1 minute per exercise
Rest whenever needed.

Level 2 (15 minutes) $1^{1}/_{2}$ minutes per exercise
Rest every second exercise.

Level 3 (20 minutes)   2 minutes per exercise
Rest every third exercise.

29	Wall Knee Lift
47	Frog Kick
25	Hip Touch
23	Kickboard Press
51	Apple Picking
16	Medley of Pulls
33	Leg Scissors
32	Bicycle Pedal
42	Posture Check
30	Back Massage

Cool-down (5 minutes)

6	Stand Tall
8	Water Kegel
5	Shoulder Shrug
9	Aqua Lunge
10	Effleurage

LAP SWIM WORKOUT 11

Swim Pointer

- Use the stroke count for the breaststroke—improves your concentration while swimming and helps you stretch out your stroke.

Reminder

Focus on a long, relaxed glide in your stroke.

Warm-up (5 minutes)

5	Shoulder Shrug
12	Breathe and Reach
8	Water Kegel
9	Aqua Lunge
1	Overhead Stretch

Main swim

Level 1 (10 minutes)

Swim 1 × 25 yards using the breaststroke stroke count.
Swim 1 × 50 yards—choose any stroke.
Rest.
Swim 1 × 25 yards using the breaststroke stroke count.
Swim 1 × 50 yards—choose any stroke.
Rest.
Swim 1 × 25 yards using the breaststroke stroke count.
Swim 1 × 50 yards—choose any stroke.
Rest.
Swim 1 × 25 yards using the breaststroke stroke count.

Level 2 (15 minutes)

    Swim 1 × 25 yards using the breaststroke stroke count.
    Swim 1 × 100 yards—choose any stroke.
    Rest.
    Swim 1 × 25 yards using the breaststroke stroke count.
    Swim 1 × 100 yards—choose any stroke.
    Rest.
    Swim 1 × 25 yards using the breaststroke stroke count.

Level 3 (20 minutes)

    Swim 1 × 50 yards using the breaststroke stroke count.
    Swim 1 × 100 yards—choose any stroke.
    Rest.
    Swim 1 × 50 yards using the breaststroke stroke count.
    Swim 1 × 100 yards—choose any stroke.
    Rest.
    Swim 1 × 50 yards using the breaststroke stroke count.
    Swim 1 × 100 yards—choose any stroke.
    Rest.
    Swim 1 × 50 yards using the breaststroke stroke count.

Cool-down (5 minutes)

3	Feet Flex
6	Stand Tall
14	Breathe and Bob
4	Water Walk/Jog
8	Water Kegel

Lap Swim Workout 12

Warm-up (5 minutes)

5	Shoulder Shrug
12	Breathe and Reach
8	Water Kegel
9	Aqua Lunge
1	Overhead Stretch

Main swim

Level 1 (10 minutes)

Swim 1 × 100 yards using varying strokes.
- 1 × 25 yards in prone float position
- 1 × 25 yards in side position
- 1 × 25 yards in back float position
- 1 × 25 yards in prone float position

Rest 1 minute.

Swim continuously for 5 minutes using the crawl stroke or the windmill backstroke.

Level 2 (15 minutes)

Swim 1 × 100 yards using varying strokes.
- 1 × 50 yards in prone float position
- 1 × 50 yards in side position

Rest 1 minute.

Swim 1 × 100 yards using varying strokes.
- 1 × 50 yards in back float position
- 1 × 50 yards in prone float position

Rest 1 minute.

Swim continuously for 5 minutes using the crawl stroke.

Rest 1 minute.

Swim 1 × 50 yards using the breaststroke.

Level 3 (20 minutes)

1 × 200 yards using varying strokes.
- 1 × 50 yards in prone float position
- 1 × 50 yards in side position
- 1 × 50 yards in back float position
- 1 × 50 yards in prone float position

Rest 1 minute.

Swim continuously for 10 minutes using the crawl stroke or the windmill backstroke.

Rest 1 minute.

Swim 1 × 200 yards using the breaststroke or the elementary backstroke.

Cool-down (5 minutes)

3	Feet Flex
6	Stand Tall
14	Breathe and Bob
4	Water Walk/Jog
8	Water Kegel

Month 8

The workouts for the eighth month of your pregnancy are designed to accommodate everyday realities during the final trimester. You are probably still carrying your usual responsibilities at home or work, but are starting to feel the need to slow down. The first of the water exercise workouts is designed for when you may want or need to keep your hair dry to save time. The water exercise and lap swim workouts concentrate on exercises that make your last weeks as comfortable as possible.

WATER EXERCISE WORKOUT 13

Warm-up (5 minutes)

15	Labor and Delivery Breathing Patterns
4	Water Walk/Jog
12	Breathe and Reach
6	Stand Tall
8	Water Kegel

Main set

Level 1 (10 minutes)	1 minute per exercise Rest whenever needed.
Level 2 (15 minutes)	1½ minutes per exercise Rest every second exercise.
Level 3 (20 minutes)	2 minutes per exercise Rest every third exercise.

Rest whenever needed—use these levels only as a guide.

- 26 Back Extension
- 34 Calf Stretch
- 37 Leg Swirl
- 19 Sport Swing
- 42 Posture Check
- 33 Leg Scissors
- 24 Circle Spray
- 16 Medley of Pulls
- 23 Kickboard Press (variation optional)
- 40 Pendulum Body Swing

Cool-down (5 minutes)

- 9 Aqua Lunge
- 15 Labor and Delivery Breathing Patterns
- 7 Pelvic Tilt
- 10 Effleurage
- 30 Back Massage

WATER EXERCISE WORKOUT 14

Warm-up (5 minutes)

- 15 Labor and Delivery Breathing Patterns
- 4 Water Walk/Jog
- 12 Breathe and Reach
- 6 Stand Tall
- 8 Water Kegel

Main set

Level 1 (10 minutes) 1 minute per exercise
Rest whenever needed.

Level 2 (15 minutes) 1$\frac{1}{2}$ minutes per exercise
Rest every second exercise.

Level 3 (20 minutes) 2 minutes per exercise
Rest every third exercise.

- 17 Arm Press
- 28 Swing and Sway
- 21 Sculling
- 47 Frog Kick
- 26 Back Extension
- 38 Double Leg Circle
- 39 Arm and Leg Reach
- 43 Deep-Water Jog
- 20 Hang 10
- 30 Back Massage

Cool-down (5 minutes)

- 9   Aqua Lunge
- 15 Labor and Delivery Breathing Patterns
- 7   Pelvic Tilt
- 10 Effleurage
- 30 Back Massage

Lap Swim Workout 13

Swim Pointer

- Focus on coordinating your exhalation with the glide phase of the breaststroke, sidestroke, or elementary backstroke.

Reminders

Rest whenever needed. Exhale completely during the glide phase. Try to concentrate and relax completely during your glide.

Warm-up (5 minutes)

11	Cleansing Breath
48	Scull and Hug
8	Water Kegel
50	Under and Over
46	Breaststroke Arm Pull

Main swim

Level 1 (10 minutes)

Swim 1 × 75 yards using the breaststroke.
Rest.
Swim 1 × 75 yards using the sidestroke.
Rest.
Swim 1 × 75 yards using the elementary backstroke.

Level 2 (15 minutes)

Swim 1 × 75 yards using the breaststroke.
Rest.
Swim 1 × 150 yards using any stroke you choose.
Rest.
Swim 1 × 75 yards using the backstroke or sidestroke.

Level 3 (20 minutes)

Swim 1 × 75 yards using the breaststroke.
Rest.
Swim 1 × 150 yards using the sidestroke.
Rest.
Swim 1 × 150 yards using the elementary backstroke.
Rest.
Swim 1 × 75 yards using any stroke you choose.

Cool-down (5 minutes)

13	Breathing With Head Circles
40	Pendulum Body Swing
11	Cleansing Breath
10	Effleurage
1	Overhead Stretch

Lap Swim Workout 14

Warm-up (5 minutes)

11	Cleansing Breath
48	Scull and Hug
8	Water Kegel
50	Under and Over
46	Breaststroke Arm Pull

Main swim

Level 1 (10 minutes)

Swim 3 × 50 yards using the crawl stroke or the backstroke with rest as needed between swims.
Swim 2 × 25 yards using the sidestroke or the breaststroke.

Level 2 (15 minutes)

Swim 3 × 100 yards using the crawl stroke or the backstroke with rest as needed between swims.
Swim 2 × 25 yards using the sidestroke.
Swim 2 × 25 yards using the breaststroke.

Level 3 (20 minutes)

Swim 2 × 100 yards using the crawl stroke or the backstroke with rest as needed between swims.
Swim 2 × 50 yards using the sidestroke.
Swim 2 × 50 yards using the breaststroke.
Swim 1 × 100 yards using the backstroke.
Swim 1 × 100 yards using the crawl stroke (optional).

Cool-down (5 minutes)

	13	Breathing With Head Circles
	40	Pendulum Body Swing
	11	Cleansing Breath
	10	Effleurage
	1	Overhead Stretch

Month 9

Most mothers-to-be find they slow up considerably during the last weeks. You can reduce your main swim time and increase your warm-up and cool-down times to about 10 minutes each.

The last workouts take into consideration that your figure has expanded. You may be practicing your exercises from your prepared childbirth class as well as stretching your leg muscles in preparation for the birth. This then is your final stretch.

WATER EXERCISE WORKOUT | 15

Warm-up (10 minutes)

	14	Breathe and Bob
	4	Water Walk/Jog
	11	Cleansing Breath
	9	Aqua Lunge
	15	Labor and Delivery Breathing Patterns

Main set

Level 1 (5 minutes)	1/2 minute per exercise Rest whenever needed.
Level 2 (10 minutes)	1 minute per exercise Rest every second exercise.
Level 3 (15 minutes)	1 1/2 minutes per exercise Rest every third exercise.

- 18 Arm Circle
- 26 Back Extension
- 28 Swing and Sway
- 21 Sculling
- 23 Kickboard Press (variation)
- 25 Hip Touch
- 16 Medley of Pulls
- 39 Arm and Leg Reach
- 29 Wall Knee Lift
- 47 Frog Kick

Cool-down (10 minutes)

- 8   Water Kegel
- 11 Cleansing Breath
- 6   Stand Tall
- 15 Labor and Delivery Breathing Patterns
- 10 Effleurage

WATER EXERCISE WORKOUT 16

Warm-up (10 minutes)

- 14 Breathe and Bob
- 4   Water Walk/Jog
- 11 Cleansing Breath
- 9   Aqua Lunge
- 15 Labor and Delivery Breathing Patterns

Main set

Level 1 (5 minutes) $1/2$ minute per exercise
                        Rest whenever needed.

Level 2 (10 minutes) 1 minute per exercise
                        Rest every second exercise.

Level 3 (15 minutes) $1^1/_2$ minutes per exercise
                        Rest every third exercise.

19	Sport Swing
25	Hip Touch
42	Posture Check
37	Leg Swirl
49	Back Flutter Kick
41	Treading
24	Circle Spray
26	Back Extension
33	Leg Scissors
47	Frog Kick

Cool-down (10 minutes)

8	Water Kegel
11	Cleansing Breath
6	Stand Tall
15	Labor and Delivery Breathing Patterns
10	Effleurage

Lap Swim Workout 15

Swim Pointer

- Remember to increase the length of your warm-up and your cool-down to 10 minutes each. This will make your workout more relaxed.

Reminders

To maintain your total workout time, decrease your main swim accordingly. Practice your cleansing breath and effleurage during your rest periods.

Warm-up (10 minutes)

Increase your warm-up time by doing exercises and then repeating the set.

- 8 Water Kegel
- 3 Feet Flex
- 5 Shoulder Shrug
- 7 Pelvic Tilt

Main swim

Level 1 (5-10 minutes)

Swim 3 minutes continuously.
Rest for 2 minutes or as needed.
Swim for 3 minutes continuously.

Level 2 (10-15 minutes)

Swim 5 minutes continuously.
Rest for 3 minutes or as needed.
Swim 5 minutes continuously.

Level 3 (15-20 minutes)

Swim 8 minutes continuously.
Rest for 3 minutes or as needed.
Swim 5 minutes continuously.

Cool-down (10 minutes)

- 34 Calf Stretch
- 9 Aqua Lunge
- 10 Effleurage
- 15 Labor and Delivery Breathing Patterns

Lap Swim Workout 16

Swim Pointer

- Focus on transition breathing.
- Increase warm-up and cool-down time.

Reminders

Review exercises in your prepared childbirth class. Stretch and strengthen inner thighs during main set.

Warm-up (10 minutes)

- 8 Water Kegel
- 9 Aqua Lunge

Add exercises of your choice.

Main swim

Level 1 (5 minutes)

Briefly swim laps, using stroke of your choice (optional).

Level 2 (10 minutes)

Swim easy laps, using a stroke of your choice, for 5 minutes. Rest when needed.

Level 3 (15 minutes)

Swim easy laps, using a stroke of your choice, for 10 minutes. Rest when needed.

Cool-down (10 minutes)

Review breathing patterns.

- 6 Stand Tall
- 8 Water Kegel
- 9 Aqua Lunge

part V

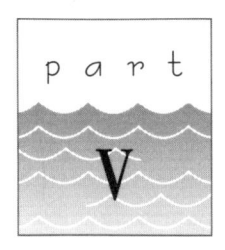

POSTPARTUM WATER FITNESS PROGRAM

Congratulations! You have just taken your part in the scheme of creation by bringing a new life into the world. Although babies are born every day, we should not allow the frequency of this event to detract from the wonder of it or from the possibilities in every baby.

Right now, however, as the mother of a newborn infant, you most likely have your sights set at closer range, asking questions like When will I be able to get into the shower? What will we be eating for dinner tonight? Or maybe, When will I be able to go back into the swimming pool? Most women at this stage are learning to balance the needs of their bodies, their newborns, and their households. Although balancing these demands is a continual process (faster for some than for others) and beyond the scope of this book, *Water Fitness During Your Pregnancy* can help in one area. Whether you're feeling great, or impatient with your physical recovery, or having bouts of postpartum depression, you can adapt the water fitness program you followed before your baby was born to help keep water fitness a pleasant and beneficial part of your life.

This part of the book outlines a postpartum water fitness program that includes activities limited during your pregnancy. Chapter 16 focuses on how-tos to help you get back in shape, including water ballet exercises, introduction to the butterfly stroke, and a 12-week postpartum water fitness program. Chapter 17 highlights expanding water activities to include your family life. It also includes Masters swimming, synchronized swim starters, water play with your newborn, and a family swim program.

POSTPARTUM DEPRESSION

Just a note about the "baby blues"—technically, postpartum depression—a common phenomenon considered to be caused by a number of factors. The physical effort of childbirth, changes in estrogen and progesterone levels, the need to take on new tasks despite fatigue from having sleep interrupted by feeding the baby, and the overwhelming sense of responsibility for the new life entrusted to her all make a woman feel very vulnerable. In addition, she has to cope with the emotions of other people adjusting to their new roles as father, older sibling, or perhaps grandparent!

For most women, the baby blues last a few days or weeks. If you acknowledge all the stresses affecting you and allow yourself to release your emotions, you will most likely find this transition time to be only temporary. After a minority of births, the blues may last more than a few weeks and these new mothers may be helped by professional counseling.

If you are going through the baby blues, make it a priority to have contact with other new mothers—friends, relatives, or neighbors who just had babies or members of an organized "new-moms" support group. Realizing that you are not the only one who has these unexpectedly negative experiences goes a long way toward alleviating fears about your own well-being.

Maintain your usual activities through the postpartum period, including physical activity once you have your doctor's OK. If you can return to the pool, physical activity can help your body cope with postpartum emotional stresses. In addition, swimming will get you out of the house, enable you to socialize with other swimmers, and help you regain your prepregnancy figure.

chapter 16

GETTING BACK IN SHAPE

You've just experienced one of humankind's most remarkable experiences—giving birth. The object of this book has been to prepare your body for labor and delivery through water fitness. Your efforts probably were rewarded and your conditioning was a great help to you during delivery. This conditioning should also help you recover more quickly.

Most women are ready to resume swimming within 4 to 6 weeks after giving birth, but you should have your doctor's approval before you start. If you had a vaginal delivery, you may have had an episiotomy to make the delivery easier. If you had a cesarean section, you may have had a bikini incision or a navel to pubic bone incision; in either case, you had abdominal surgery, and your muscles need time to heal before you return to the water. Lochia, a vaginal discharge following delivery, is a natural drainage of the uterus that lasts approximately 6 weeks. Wait until the discharge has ceased before beginning the program. After you've received your doctor's OK, you're ready to take the plunge.

Postpartum Water Exercise Guidelines

These general tips will be helpful during your postpartum period:

- Be safe rather than sorry—return to the water only with your obstetrician's go-ahead. You must be completely recovered from delivery before starting your postpartum exercise program. Your doctor will advise you when the healing process is complete.
- It may take a year to completely return to your prepregnancy figure and weight. This may be a slow process, but in the long run, it is

better to move gradually toward your former figure and weight than crash diet in order to lose the weight all at once.
- Start exercising gently and gradually increase the workouts. (The swim program is set up specifically for gradual progression.)
- Your ligaments remain soft for approximately 5 months after the birth. Take care not to overstretch.
- In particular, do not overwork your abdominal muscles—they have just been under a lot of stress.
- Continue to swim with a supporting bra while your breasts are still enlarged.
- Continue to pay attention to maintaining good posture in and out of the water.
- The Kegel exercise is as important as before your delivery. Be sure to include it in your workouts.
- Think about whether you would prefer to swim in a facility with child care available, or whether you would benefit from having your water fitness time completely to yourself.
- To regain your prepregnancy figure, pay special attention to your buttocks; upper, outer, and inner thighs; abdomen; chest; and waist.
- Don't be discouraged if you tire easily. You've assumed a new role as a mother, and you'll have to adjust other aspects of your life to it. This may take some time, but *don't* get discouraged.
- If you find that you're having some difficulty swimming, increase the time you spend on the warm-up and cool-down.
- You may have to give yourself a mental boost to keep water fitness in your schedule, but don't give up—the benefits of swimming are worth the extra effort.
- Swimming is good for the inner you and the outer you. Return to the basics and work your way up.
- Try to set aside a specific amount of time to devote to swimming. Ask your partner to join you—the baby will join you later.
- The postpartum workouts provide a choice of water exercises. Select those that are appropriate for your recovery progress, comfort level, and fitness goals.
- Explore other forms of swimming activity, such as the Masters swimming program, a low-key competitive program in which you can participate for a lifetime.

So—here you are, Mom. Enjoy your swim!

Water Ballet Exercises

Water ballet, now known as the sport of synchronized swimming, is rhythmically performed swimming skills synchronized to music. In

Europe, where it began, it was also known as "ornamental swimming." The artistic nature of this aquatic activity is often compared to figure skating because it combines the benefits of an art form with the benefits of a sport. Synchronized swimming is now an Olympic sport—it has come a long way since Esther Williams's time.

After your pregnancy, you can enjoy the benefits of this creative and graceful water activity. You'll use skills from your WET exercises as the basis for basic synchronized swimming skills, combining them with your swim strokes to create beautiful movements and sequences in the water (see Table 16.1). You will find that toning and tightening your muscles, especially the abdominals, can be a beautiful experience as well as a beneficial one.

Let there be music! You can practice your movements to piped-in music, or even listen to music with a waterproof tape player or radio. Experiment with different types, tempos, and moods to create your own set of movements in a water routine.

Synchronized swimming can be an addition to or an extension of your swimming workouts during and after your pregnancy. For example, you can combine these swim stroke variations in different ways to create your own routine.

- Alternate the crawl and backstroke every three strokes.
- Alternate the sidestroke with the breaststroke, changing sides.

Table 16.1 Suggested Swimming Stroke Variations for Water Ballet

Stroke	Head	Arm motion	Leg movement
Crawl	Head remains forward and out of water	Straight-arm recovery	Bent-knee flutter kick underwater
Breaststroke	Head remains out of water, turn head at the catch after each stroke	Hands splash on extension	Flutter kick underwater
Backstroke	Chin up; head remains still	Windmill backstroke or salute stroke	Slow bent-knee flutter kick underwater
Sidestroke	Head remains still or alternates moving forward and back	Alternate overarm with regular arm pull	Alternate scissors with flutter kicks on glide

- Combine all the strokes while moving in the same direction—one breaststroke, one sidestroke, one backstroke, one crawl stroke, one breaststroke.
- Create your own combinations.

A final note: a basic component for executing and performing many of these synchronized swimming movements is sculling, the figure-eight motion used in treading. Sculling allows you to move in different directions, and it supports your body in different positions. Five sample water ballet exercises follow that you can incorporate into your postpartum program.

52

MARLIN TURN

Benefits
Tones the entire body.

Starting Position
Begin in a back float (layout) position with your arms extended at shoulder level. Your face, hips, thighs, and feet are at the water's surface.

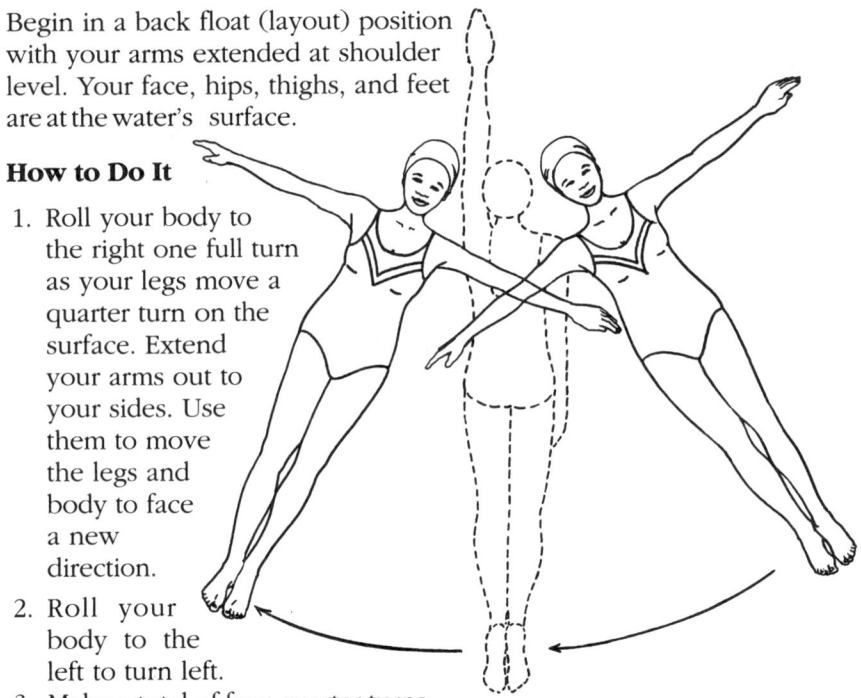

How to Do It
1. Roll your body to the right one full turn as your legs move a quarter turn on the surface. Extend your arms out to your sides. Use them to move the legs and body to face a new direction.
2. Roll your body to the left to turn left.
3. Make a total of four quarter turns (90° each) as close as possible to the surface of the water.

Exercise Tip
- Your face may be above or below the surface as you complete each turn.

Tuck Turn

Benefits

Tones entire body, especially the abdomen. This position can be beneficial in relieving lower-back pain.

Starting Position

Begin in the back layout position.

How to Do It

1. Bring your knees toward your chest, keeping shins close to the water's surface.
2. Remaining in the tuck position, turn your body 360°, pushing the water by turning your palms sideways in the opposite direction, keeping your face above the water.
3. Repeat, going the other way.

Exercise Tip

- As you drop your hips, bring your shins parallel to the surface of the water. Don't let your knees pop up.

CLAM

Benefits

Tones abdomen and stretches lower leg muscles.

Starting Position

Begin in a back layout position.

How to Do It

1. With your arms, create a downward and overhead circular movement as the hips pike, drawing your straightened legs to your chest.
2. Move your hands out of the water to approach your feet before submerging.

Exercise Tips

- As your abdomen increases in strength, pike your hips more, trying to touch your hands to your feet.
- Remember to stretch and point your toes.

BENT-KNEE MARCHING STEP

Benefits

Tones arms and abdomen. This total-body exercise is especially good for postpartum shape-up. Sculling faster for tone and strength helps the arms, the chest, the waist, the legs—it's wonderful!

Starting Position

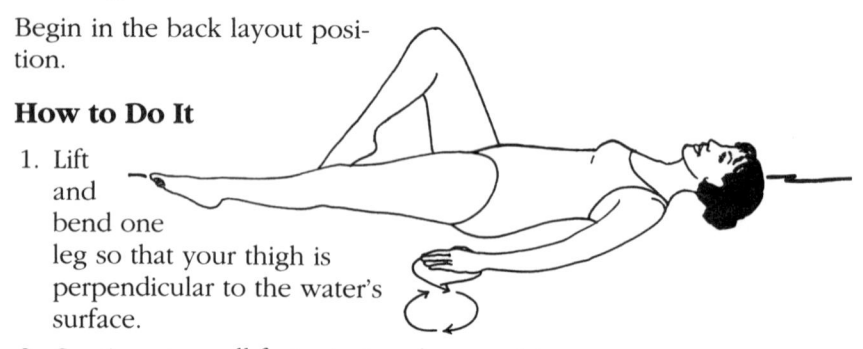

Begin in the back layout position.

How to Do It

1. Lift and bend one leg so that your thigh is perpendicular to the water's surface.
2. Continue to scull faster just under your hips.

Exercise Tip

- Try moving in a headfirst direction by flexing your wrists and pointing your fingers upward slightly as you scull.

Variations

- Try alternately bending both legs.
- If you are having difficulty keeping the straight leg on the surface, place it on the pool's edge or have someone support you lightly under your ankle.

Shark Circle

Benefits

Stretches your sides and abdomen.

Starting Position

Begin in a back layout position. Turn to either side to assume a side layout position with the top arm extended overhead. The arm should be next to your ear, close to the water's surface.

How to Do It

1. Scull with your lower arm to move your body in a complete circle on the surface.
2. Complete your Shark Circle by resuming your back layout position.

Exercise Tips

- For an extra boost for propulsion, add a small flutter kick.
- Keep your back arched evenly throughout your circle.

Variation

- Reverse direction.

Butterfly Stroke

Perhaps you're saying to yourself, "Let's skip this stroke." But wait—The exciting, graceful butterfly stroke is not beyond your abilities.

The arm motion for the butterfly is similar to the S-shaped pull crawl motion, done using both arms simultaneously with an over-water recovery. Because the arms move at the same time, there is no body roll. The leg motion is called the dolphin kick—it is similar to the flutter kick except that the legs move together.

The butterfly stroke breathing pattern is similar to that used with the breaststroke, in which your head and shoulders rise as you pull. Coordinating these components produces a wavelike body motion that resembles the diving motion of a dolphin. There is no denying that the butterfly is a strenuous stroke, but it can be done! So try it!

Body Position

Begin in a prone streamlined body position.

Arm Motion

For the *catch*, extend your arms underwater, shoulder-width apart, thumbs downward (see Figure 16.6). *Pull* your arms outward and downward, beginning a keyhole arm pattern. Then bring your hands together under your abdomen, near your waist, elbows bent about 90°, and press the water backward toward your feet. When your arms are almost fully extended with your hands near your hips, the *recovery* begins. Your arms recover out of the water, with elbows leading as they swing forward to the catch or starting position.

Leg Motion

The dolphin kick is used for the butterfly stroke (see Figure 16.7 on page 188). Your legs move up and down, as in the flutter kick, but in unison. To create a wavelike body motion, bring your hips up, with your buttocks breaking the surface of the water as your legs kick on the downbeat. On the upbeat, your feet should barely break the surface.

Breathing

Take your breath at the end of the arm pull, just as your arms are beginning to recover. Lift your chin forward just enough to take a breath. Then lower your head immediately to exhale and finish your recovery, bringing your arms back to the catch position.

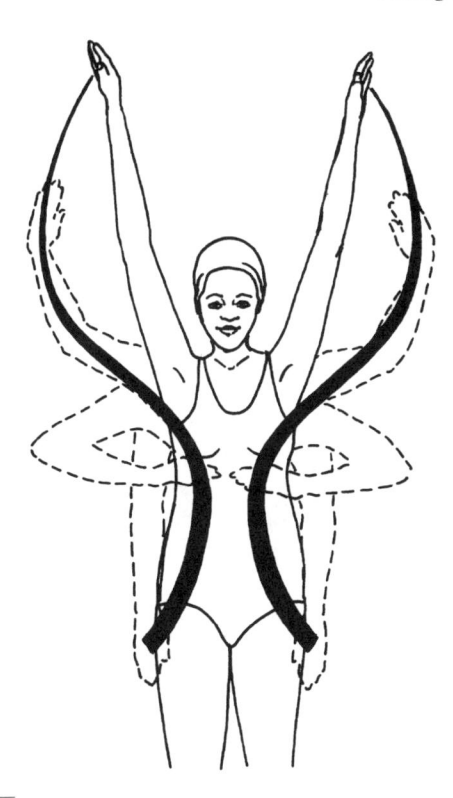

Figure 16.6 The butterfly keyhole pull.

Stroke Coordination

Although the butterfly is normally done with a two-beat kick per arm stroke, it's easier to learn to coordinate your arm and leg motions by starting with a single-beat kick per arm stroke (see Figure 16.8 on page 189). Begin in an extended prone float position, arms extended underwater, shoulder-width apart for the *catch*. Bend your legs as you bend your arms for the *pull*, and straighten your legs as you bring your arms above the water for the *recovery*. Lift your head for a breath as your shoulders rise during your pull.

Push-Off

The butterfly stroke consists of simultaneous arm and leg motions (like the breaststroke with an over-water recovery). The push-off for butterfly is also similar to the breaststroke push-off. Stand with your back against the pool wall, extend your arms in front of you, and straighten your legs.

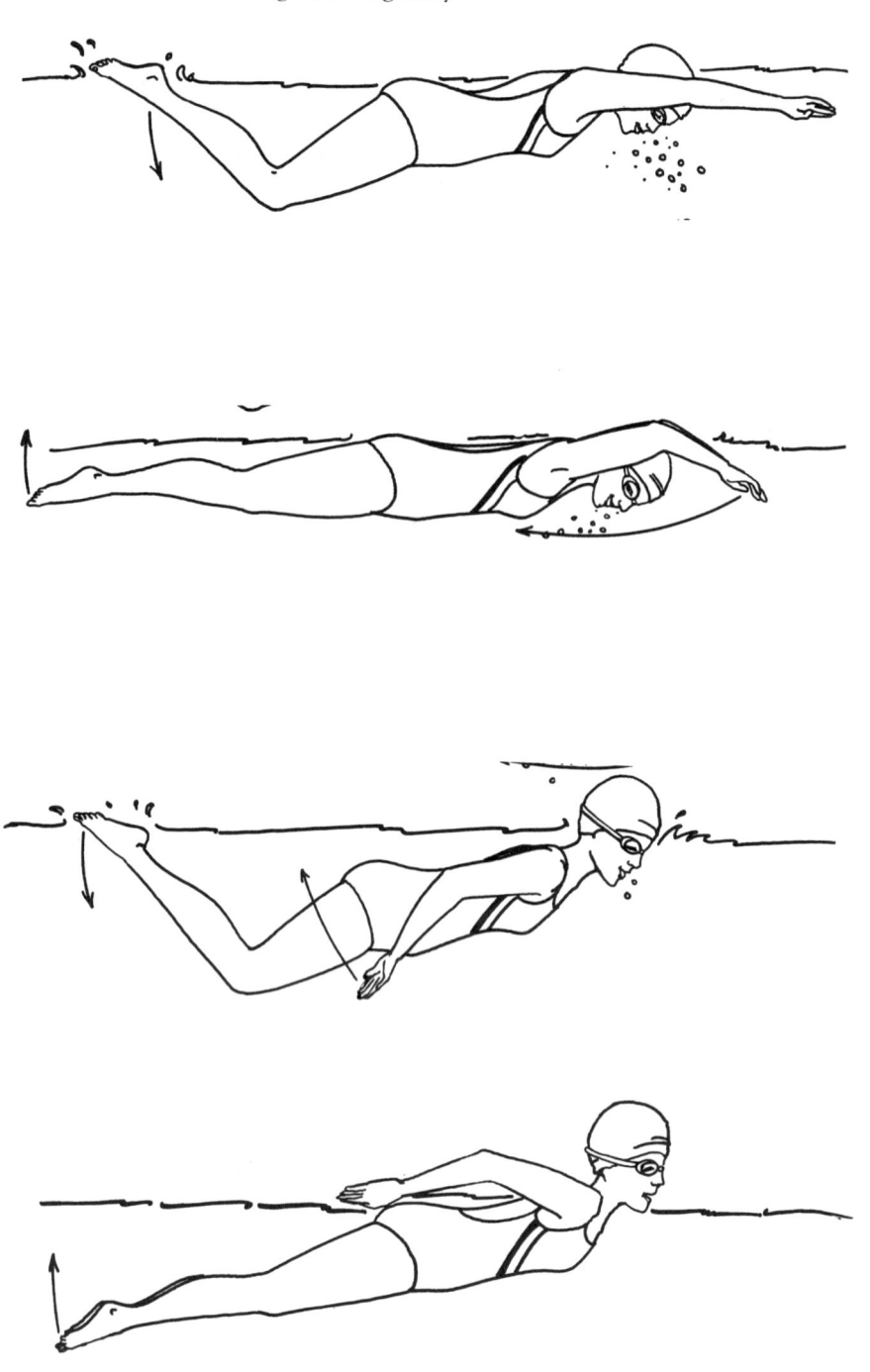

Figure 16.7 The double-beat butterfly dolphin kick.

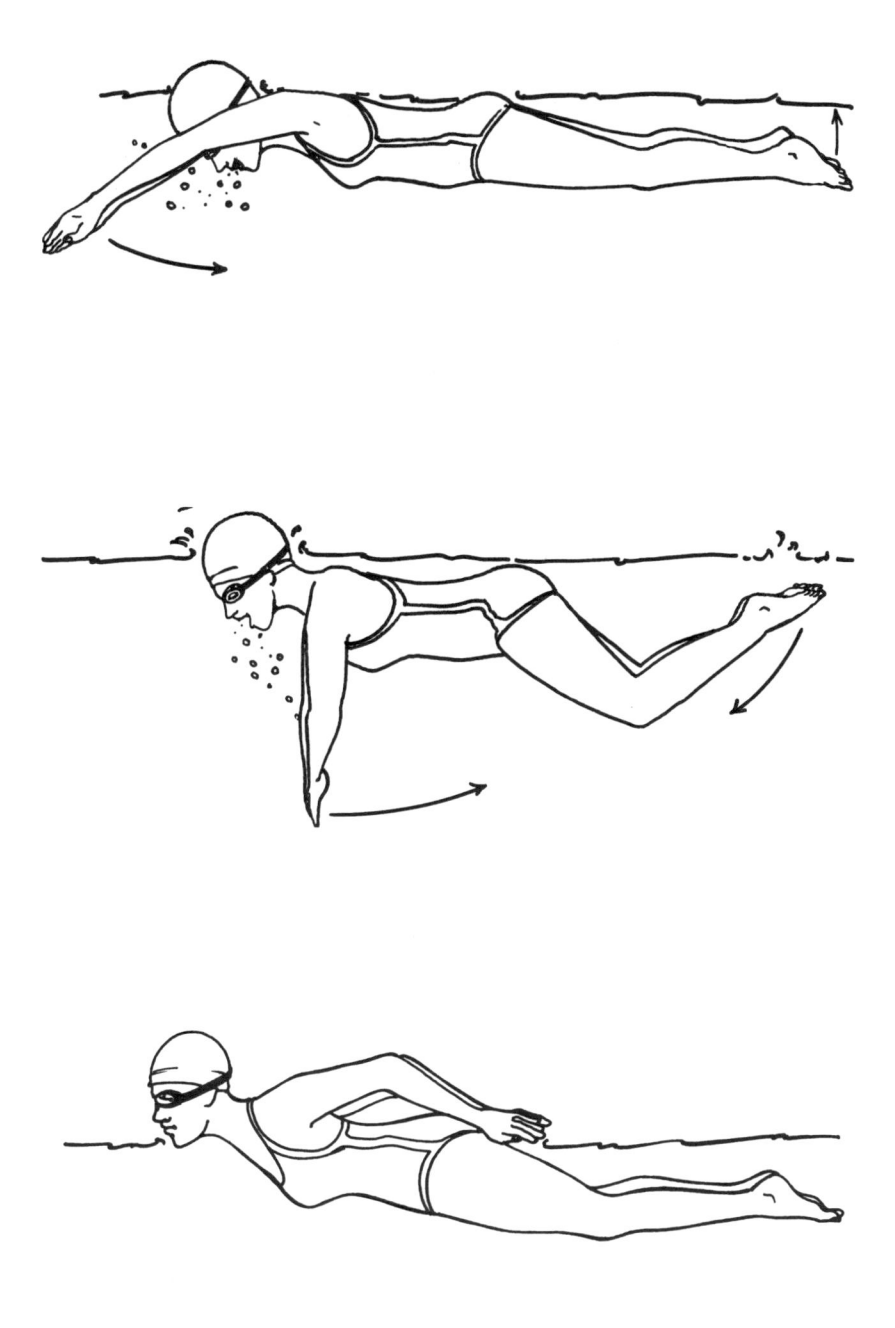

Figure 16.8 The single-beat butterfly dolphin kick.

Turns

The butterfly turn is also similar to the breaststroke turn. Glide into the wall with your arms extended in front of you. Touch the wall with both hands at the water's surface. As you touch the wall, inhale immediately and turn toward one side by releasing that hand (e.g., turn to left, extend left hand). Then extend that same hand the opposite direction. Finish the turn as a crawl open turn by bringing the other arm to join the forward arm. Push off by straightening your legs and assuming the prone streamlined body position.

Butterfly Tips

- The keyhole butterfly arm stroke is similar to the freestyle S-shaped pull, with your arms moving simultaneously, but without a body roll. The right arm traces a reverse *S* pattern of a question mark while the left arm traces an *S* pattern or reverse question mark.
- Try "flutterfly"—a combination of the butterfly and crawl stroke. Use the crawl arm motion with the dolphin kick or the butterfly pull with the flutter kick.
- Coordinate the butterfly arm motion first with the single dolphin kick, then the two-beat kick.
- To get the wavelike dolphin movement you can experiment using fins. You can also use fins to develop more propulsion, power, and flexibility. Fins are not cheating!
- Begin the butterfly at short distances and work up to a maximum distance of 25 yards at any one time.
- *Reminder.* If you have any back concern, substitute other strokes for the butterfly in your postpartum workouts.

57

DOLPHIN SIT AND KICK

Benefits

Strengthens and tones abdominal muscles while allowing you to practice the butterfly's simultaneous leg motion.

Equipment

Fins (optional)

Starting Position

Sit at pool's edge with your knees bent.

How to Do It

1. Drop your heels simultaneously to touch the wall.
2. Then simultaneously straighten your knees and lift your legs to the water's surface, with your toes pointed.

Variation

- For extra resistance, do this exercise with fins, preferably small flexible fins. This variation will also help strengthen leg muscles.

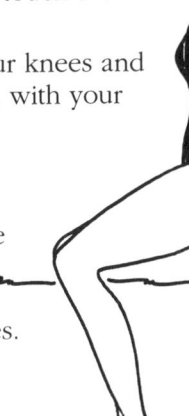

58

ROPE JUMP

Benefits

Simulates coordination of butterfly stroke. This is a total-body exercise that strengthens the arm and abdominal muscles.

Starting Position

Stand in chest-deep water, with feet hip-width apart.

How to Do It

1. Simulate jumping rope. Keep feet together and lift arms out of the water overhead.
2. Clear "rope" with your feet as arms pass your thighs and move behind you.

Variation

- Then add a second knee bend just as arms recover to simulate two-beat (double-beat) kick.

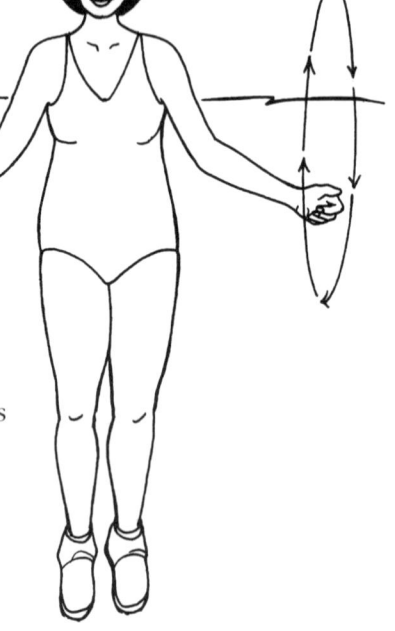

Postpartum Workouts

A 12-week progressive swim program with suggested workouts for the postpartum period follows. It includes synchronized swimming (water ballet) and swim skills, including the butterfly stroke.

During this part of the program, you move progressively from easy workouts to more challenging ones as you recover. After the 12-week program, you'll be prepared to go on to a more energetic swimming program.

The postpartum program is similar to the pregnancy program in that each exercise session starts with a 5-minute warm-up, proceeds to a main swim of 10 to 20 minutes, and finishes with a 5-minute cool-down. Again, you can select from three levels of main swim sets, depending on your fitness level and recovery from delivery. Don't hesitate to change from level to level in the main swim—let your health and fitness be your guide, and listen to your body.

The workouts include an introduction to synchronized swimming skills because synchronized swimming is a terrific conditioner, as well as lots of fun. Synchronized swimming employs all the muscles of the body, develops grace and coordination, and is a great aerobic exercise. It also helps burn calories. As you become more fit and more skilled, you'll be able to progress from water ballet to synchronized swimming exercises that use more challenging movements and patterns. This is a great way to expand your swimming repertoire.

WEEK 1

Swim Pointer

- Use this workout to get back into a swim routine and to enjoy the relaxing benefits of the water.

Reminders

Are you ready? Check with your doctor for the go-ahead to resume your swims. Listen to your body.

Warm-up (5 minutes)

14	Breathe and Bob
8	Water Kegel

Medley of water exercises: Choose three other water exercises, and rest after each one.

Main swim

Level 1 (10 minutes)	Swim, using a variety of strokes. Rest as needed.
Level 2 (15 minutes)	Swim, using a variety of strokes. Rest as needed.
Level 3 (20 minutes)	Swim, using a variety of strokes. Rest as needed.

Cool-down (5 minutes)

20	Hang 10
41	Treading

Choose three other water exercises.

WEEK 2

Swim Pointers

- Review sculling and synchronized swimming techniques.
- Use the layout position and the Marlin Turn.

Reminder

Pay attention to your swim stroke technique. This will be helpful for getting "back in the swim" and for muscle toning.

Warm-up (5 minutes)

14 Breathe and Bob
41 Treading
Choose three other water exercises.

Main swim

Level 1 (10 minutes)

Swim for 3 minutes continuously.
Rest.
Scull 2 × 25 yards using the elementary backstroke.
Rest.
From your back layout position, do two Marlin Turns to the right and to the left.

Level 2 (15 minutes)

Swim for 5 minutes continuously.
Rest.
Scull 1 × 25 yards.
Rest.
Swim 1 × 25 yards elementary backstroke.
From your back layout position, do Marlin Turns to the right and left.

Level 3 (20 minutes)

Swim for 10 minutes continuously, varying your strokes and resting as needed.
Rest.
Scull 1 × 25 yards.
Rest.
Scull 1 × 25 yards.
From your back layout position, try your Marlin Turns to the right and to the left. Then do two turns continuously.

Cool-down (5 minutes)

41 Treading
8 Water Kegel
Choose two water exercises.
52 Marlin Turn

WEEK 3

Swim Pointers

- Review skills for the various backstrokes.
- Practice tuck position.

Reminder

Rotate your shoulders while doing the windmill backstroke. Remember that the sit-up position is similar to your tuck position.

Warm-up (5 minutes)

14	Breathe and Bob
27	Modified Sit-Up
8	Water Kegel

Choose two other water exercises.

Main swim

Level 1 (10 minutes)

Swim continuously for 5 minutes—include all backstrokes.
Rest.
1 × 25 yards sculling in tuck position.
Rest.
1 × 50 yards backstroke of your choice (use a half turn in tuck position at the wall).
Rest.
1 × 25 yards sculling in tuck position.
Rest.
Practice tuck turns to the right and left.

Level 2 (15 minutes)

1 × 25 yards sculling.
Rest.
1 × 25 yards sculling.
Rest.
Swim continuously for 7 minutes. Alternate every other lap on your back.
Rest.
Practice tuck turns to the right and left.
Rest.
Swim a backstroke medley of these strokes:
- 1 × 25 yards sculling
- 1 × 25 yards elementary backstroke
- 1 × 25 yards windmill backstroke
- 1 × 25 backstroke choice

Level 3 (20 minutes)

1 × 25 yards sculling. Begin in tuck position.
Rest.
1 × 50 yards backstroke.
Rest.
1 × 25 yards sculling. Begin in tuck position.
Swim continuously for 10 minutes, with every other lap on your back.
Rest.
Practice tuck turns to the right and left.
Swim a backstroke medley of these strokes:
- 1 × 25 yards sculling
- 1 × 25 yards elementary backstroke
- 1 × 25 yards backstroke
- 1 × 25 backstroke choice

Cool-down (5 minutes)

52 Marlin Turn
41 Treading
14 Breathe and Bob

WEEK 4

Swim Pointers

- Review variations of the sidestroke.
- Practice the Marlin Turn in both directions.

Reminder

The sidestroke has eight variations, two arm variations and two leg variations on both sides.

Warm-up (5 minutes)

14	Breathe and Bob
16	Medley of Pulls
8	Water Kegel
52	Marlin Turn

Main swim

Level 1 (10 minutes)

Swim continuously for 7 minutes, including sidestroke variations.
Rest.
Swim 1 × 50 yards using your choice of backstroke.
Practice Marlin Turns to the right and left.

Level 2 (15 minutes)

Swim continuously for 10 minutes, including sidestroke variations.
Rest.
Swim 1 × 50 yards using your choice of backstroke.
Practice Marlin Turns to the right and left.

Level 3 (20 minutes)

Swim continuously for 12 minutes, including sidestroke variations.

Rest.

Swim 1 × 100 yards using a backstroke medley of these strokes:

  1 × 25 yards sculling
  1 × 25 yards elementary backstroke
  1 × 25 yards windmill backstroke
  1 × 25 yards backstroke (choice)

Practice Marlin Turns to the right and left.

Cool-down (5 minutes)

  53 Tuck Turn
  41 Treading (alternate with float position)
     Choose three other water exercises.

WEEK 5

Swim Pointers

- Review and practice butterfly stroke skills.
- Learn and practice the Clam in a pike position.
- Timed swim: Swim 50 yards as fast as you can, and record your time. Track your progress by maintaining a record of your times.

Reminders

Remember, the butterfly arm motion is similar to the crawl S-shaped pull, except that your arms move forward simultaneously in the butterfly rather than alternately as in the crawl.

When doing the Clam, try to keep your legs straight.

Warm-up (5 minutes)

- 14 Breathe and Bob
- 18 Arm Circle
- 8 Water Kegel

Choose three other warm-up exercises.

Main swim

Level 1 (10 minutes)

Swim 1 × 25 yards using the breaststroke.
Rest.
Swim 1 × 25 yards using an easy crawl.
Swim 3 × 25 yards using your choice of stroke. Vary strokes. Rest 30 seconds between swims.
Rest.
Swim 1 × 50 yards using a crawl stroke in a timed swim.

Level 2 (15 minutes)

Swim 1 × 25 yards of the breaststroke.
Swim 1 × 25 yards with an easy crawl.
Rest.
Swim 3 × 100 yards, varying your strokes. Rest 30 seconds between swims.
Rest.
Swim 1 × 50 yards using a crawl stroke in a timed swim.

Level 3 (20 minutes)

Swim 1 × 25 yards using the breaststroke.
Swim 1 × 25 yards using an easy crawl.
Rest.
Swim 3 × 150 yards, varying your strokes. Rest 30 seconds between swims.
Rest.
Swim 1 × 50 yards using the crawl stroke in a timed swim.

Cool-down (5 minutes)

- 41 Treading (alternate with float position)
- 54 Clam

Choose three other water exercises.

WEEK 6

Swim Pointers

- Practice the dolphin kick for the butterfly stroke.
- Learn the Shark Circle synchronized swimming exercise.
- Apply the pyramid training technique to your swims.

Reminders

Keep your legs moving together for the dolphin kick. Combine the crawl arm motion with the dolphin kick.

Warm-up (5 minutes)

14	Breathe and Bob
7	Pelvic Tilt
25	Hip Touch
56	Shark Circle

Main swim

Level 1 (10 minutes)

Swim 1 × 25 yards using the dolphin kick.

Rest.

Swim 1 × 25 yards using the crawl stroke with the dolphin kick.

Do a pyramid swim, resting 30 seconds between these swims:

- 1 × 25 yards
- 1 × 50 yards
- 1 × 100 yards
- 1 × 50 yards
- 1 × 25 yards

Level 2 (15 minutes)

Swim 1 × 25 yards using the dolphin kick.

Rest.

Swim 1 × 25 yards using the crawl stroke with the dolphin kick.

Do a pyramid swim, resting 30 seconds between these swims:

1 × 50 yards
1 × 75 yards
1 × 100 yards
1 × 75 yards
1 × 50 yards

Rest.

Swim 1 × 25 yards using the dolphin kick.

Swim 1 × 25 yards using the crawl stroke with the dolphin kick.

Level 3 (20 minutes)

Swim 1 × 25 yards using the dolphin kick.

Rest.

Swim 1 × 25 yards using the crawl stroke with the dolphin kick.

Do a pyramid swim, resting 30 seconds between these swims:

1 × 50 yards
1 × 100 yards
1 × 150 yards
1 × 100 yards
1 × 50 yards

Rest.

Swim 1 × 25 yards using the dolphin kick.

Swim 1 × 25 yards using the crawl stroke with the dolphin kick.

Cool-down (5 minutes)

41	Treading (alternate with float position)
56	Shark Circle (to the right and left)
52	Marlin Turn
8	Water Kegel

WEEK 7

Swim Pointers

- Practice the keyhole butterfly arm motion.
- Incorporate a kick-pull-swim set like the ones suggested in the following sets into your workout.
- Coordinate the butterfly stroke components.

Reminder

Combine the butterfly arm motion with the dolphin kick. Use fins (optional) for greater propulsion.

Warm-up (5 minutes)

- 8 Water Kegel
- 56 Shark Circle
    Choose two total-body exercises.
- 58 Rope Jump

Main swim

Level 1 (10 minutes)

Swim 1 × 75 yards using a kick-pull-swim butterfly incorporating these elements:
- 1 × 25 yards dolphin kick
- 1 × 25 yards butterfly arm motion
- 1 × 25 yards combining butterfly arm motion with dolphin kick.

Rest.

Swim 1 × 75 yards using a kick-pull-swim crawl stroke incorporating these elements:
- 1 × 25 yards flutter kick
- 1 × 25 yards crawl arm motion
- 1 × 25 yards crawl stroke.

Rest.

Level 1 *(continued)*

Swim 1 × 75 yards using a kick-pull-swim set made up of your choice of stroke.

Swim 1 × 25 yards at an easy pace using your choice of stroke.

Level 2 (15 minutes)

Swim 1 × 75 yards using a kick-pull-swim butterfly incorporating these elements:
- 1 × 25 yards dolphin kick
- 1 × 25 yards butterfly arm motion
- 1 × 25 yards combining butterfly arm motion with dolphin kick

Rest.

Swim 1 × 150 yards using a kick-pull-swim crawl stroke incorporating these elements:
- 1 × 50 yards flutter kick
- 1 × 50 yards crawl arm pull
- 1 × 50 yards crawl stroke

Rest.

Swim 1 × 75 yards using a kick-pull-swim set made up of your choice of stroke.

Swim 1 × 50 yards at an easy pace using your choice of stroke.

Level 3 (20 minutes)

Swim 1 × 75 yards using a kick-pull-swim butterfly incorporating these elements:
- 1 × 25 yards dolphin kick
- 1 × 25 yards butterfly arm pull
- 1 × 25 yards combining butterfly arm pull with dolphin kick.

Rest.

Swim 1 × 25 yards using a kick-pull-swim crawl stroke incorporating these elements:
- 1 × 75 yards flutter kick
- 1 × 75 yards crawl arm pull
- 1 × 75 yards crawl stroke

Rest.

Swim 1 × 150 yards using a kick-pull-swim set made up of your choice of stroke.

Swim 1 × 50 yards at an easy pace using your choice of stroke.

Cool-down (5 minutes)

20 Hang 10
41 Treading (alternate with float position)
21 Sculling
   Choose two middle-body exercises.

~~~~~~~~~~~~~~~~~~~~~~~~

WEEK 8

Swim Pointers

- Practice the butterfly stroke.
- Combine an individual medley of swim strokes.
- Learn the Bent-Knee Marching Step.

Reminders

The individual medley consists of the butterfly, backstroke, breaststroke, and crawl.

Practice the Bent-Knee Marching Step by first facing the wall and resting your foot on the edge, step, or ladder for support. Keep your leg straight.

Warm-up (5 minutes)

 4 Water Walk/Jog
26 Back Extension (If you have a back concern, replace this exercise with exercise 29, Wall Knee Lift.)
27 Modified Sit-Up
16 Medley of Pulls

Main swim

Level 1 (10 minutes)

Swim 1 × 100 yards using an individual medley incorporating these strokes:
- 1 × 25 yards butterfly
- 1 × 25 yards backstroke of your choice
- 1 × 25 yards breaststroke
- 1 × 25 yards crawl stroke

Rest.

Swim 1 × 100 yards using the stroke of your choice.

Rest.

Swim 1 × 100 yards using an individual medley.

Level 2 (15 minutes)

Swim 1 × 100 yards using an individual medley incorporating these strokes:
- 1 × 25 yards butterfly
- 1 × 25 yards backstroke of your choice
- 1 × 25 yards breaststroke
- 1 × 25 yards crawl stroke

Rest.

Swim 1 × 200 yards using the stroke of your choice.

Rest.

Swim 1 x 100 yards using an individual medley.

Level 3 (20 minutes)

Swim 1 × 100 yards using an individual medley incorporating these strokes:
- 1 × 25 yards butterfly
- 1 × 25 yards backstroke
- 1 × 25 yards breaststroke
- 1 × 25 yards crawl stroke

Rest.

Swim 1 × 200 yards using the stroke of your choice.

Rest.

Swim 1 × 100 yards using an individual medley.

Rest.

Swim 1 × 200 yards using the stroke of your choice.

Rest.

Swim 1 × 100 yards using an individual medley.

Cool-down (5 minutes)

57	Dolphin Sit and Kick
8	Water Kegel
35	Wall Walk
52	Marlin Turn

WEEK 9

Swim Pointers

- Apply interval training to your workout (see p. 136).
- Review Clam, Tuck Turn, and Shark Circle.

Reminder

Review push-offs and turns for all strokes.

Warm-up (5 minutes)

8	Water Kegel
46	Breaststroke Arm Pull
37	Leg Swirl
54	Clam

Main swim

Level 1 (10 minutes)

Swim 1 × 150 yards using the stroke of your choice.
Rest.
Swim 3 × 50 yards crawl on 2 minutes.

Level 2 (15 minutes)

Swim 3 × 50 yards using the crawl on 1:30 minutes.
Swim 1 × 200 yards using the stroke of your choice.
Rest.
Swim 3 × 50 yards using the crawl on 1:30 minutes.

Level 3 (20 minutes)

Swim 1 × 100 yards using an individual medley.
Rest.
Swim 4 × 50 yards using the crawl on 1 minute.
Rest.
Swim 1 × 200 yards using the stroke of your choice.
Rest.
Swim 4 × 50 yards using the crawl on 1 minute.

Cool-down (5 minutes)

52	Marlin Turn
56	Shark Circle
34	Calf Stretch
25	Hip Touch

WEEK 10

Swim Pointers

- Review Bent-Knee Marching Step.
- Practice sidestroke variations.

Reminders

Alternately bend and straighten each leg to practice Bent-Knee Marching Step.

Warm-up (5 minutes)

50	Over and Under
51	Apple Picking
40	Pendulum Body Swing
21	Sculling
54	Clam

Main swim

Level 1 (10 minutes)

Swim 1 × 100 yards sidestroke medley with these variations on both sides.
   1 × 25 yards regular arm and regular scissors kick
   1 × 25 yards regular arm motion and inverted kick
   1 × 25 yards overarm variation and regular kick
   1 × 25 yards overarm variation and inverted kick
Rest.
Swim 3 × 50 yards using the crawl stroke on 1:45 minutes.
Rest.
Swim 1 × 100 yards at an easy pace using your choice of strokes.

Level 2 (15 minutes)

Swim 1 × 100 yards using a sidestroke medley with variations on both sides.
Rest.
Swim 3 × 50 yards using a crawl stroke on 1:30 minutes.
Rest.
Swim 1 × 200 yards using the stroke of your choice.
Rest.
Swim 2 × 50 yards using the crawl stroke on 1:20 minutes.

Level 3 (20 minutes)

Swim 1 × 100 yards using a sidestroke medley with variations on both sides.
Swim 5 × 50 yards crawl stroke on 1 minute.
Swim 1 × 300 yards using the stroke of your choice.
Swim 2 × 50 yards on 50 seconds.

Cool-down (5 minutes)

   31   Flutter Kick
   20   Hang 10
   41   Treading
    8   Water Kegel

WEEK 11

Swim Pointers

- Review turns and push-off.
- Try a continuous swim.

Reminders

For breaststroke and butterfly, touch the wall with two hands. For crawl, backstroke, and sidestroke, touch the wall with leading hand.

Warm-up (5 minutes)

   8   Water Kegel
  27 Modified Sit-Up

Choose three other exercises.

Main swim

Level 1 (10 minutes)

Swim continuously for 5 minutes, varying your strokes. Rest.
Swim 3 × 50 yards on 1:45 minutes.

Level 2 (15 minutes)

Swim continuously for 8 minutes, varying your strokes. Rest.
Swim 3 × 50 yards on 1:20 minutes.

Level 3 (20 minutes)

Swim continuously for 12 minutes, varying your strokes. Rest.
Swim 5 × 50 yards on 1 minute.

Cool-down (5 minutes)

  49 Back Flutter Kick
  16 Medley of Pulls
      Choose three other exercises.

WEEK 12

Swim Pointers

- Combine water ballet synchronized swimming figures and stroke variations to form a pattern.
- Time yourself swimming 1 × 50 yards.

Reminders

Smooth, graceful movements are basic both for swimming and for synchronized swimming.
Vary strokes for continuous swim.

Warm-up (5 minutes)

  8 Water Kegel
     1 x 50 yards easy swim
     Synchronized swimming stroke variations and skills

Main swim

Level 1 (10 minutes)

Swim continuously for 5 minutes.
Rest.
Swim 2 × 25 yards using a synchronized swimming pattern that combines two figures with two stroke variations. Repeat the sequence for the entire lap.
Rest between lengths.
Swim 1 × 50 yards using the crawl stroke in a timed swim.

Level 2 (15 minutes)

Swim continuously for 8 minutes.
Rest.
Swim 2 × 25 yards using a synchronized swimming pattern that combines three figures with three stroke variations. Repeat the sequence for the entire lap.
Rest.
Swim 1 × 50 yards using the crawl stroke in a timed swim.

Level 3 (20 minutes)

Swim continuously for 12 minutes.
Rest.
Swim 1 × 50 yards using a synchronized swimming pattern that combines three or more figures with three or more stroke variations. Repeat the sequence for the entire lap.
Rest.
Swim 1 × 50 yards using the crawl stroke in a timed swim.

Cool-down (5 minutes)

	Medley of Kicks (alternate flutter, dolphin, frog, and scissors kicks)
16	Medley of Pulls
	Choose three other exercises.

chapter 17

EXPANDING YOUR WATER EXERCISE PROGRAM

You can continue your water fitness program in many ways, including aquatic fitness classes, Masters swimming, and synchronized swimming. Introducing your baby to the water and playing in the water with your newborn is a special time. If you have other children, many family swim opportunities and programs are available.

This chapter highlights how to expand your water fitness program and offers sources for more information.

Masters Swimming

Now that you're back in the swim, broaden your swimming horizons. You can choose anything from water exercises to a progressive fitness program.

If you have used the swim logs in this book during and after your pregnancy, you may continue to use them to log your swim distances and/or water exercise workout time. Another way to keep track of your lap swimming is to use the chart in Figure 17.1, which has space to record each quarter-mile you swim, up to 50 miles.

If you've followed any part of the postpartum program in this book, you may have developed a new fitness outlook, and you may wish to use your new swim skills in a low-key competitive swim program known as Masters swimming.

There's more to Masters swimming than just laps. The main purpose of Masters swimming is to promote physical fitness. Competitions are organized so you compete with women within your 5-year age bracket (e.g., 19-24, 25-29, 30-34, 35-39, 40-44, 45-49, etc.). You can choose from a variety of distances and strokes—different strokes for different folks clearly applies to this situation. Competition can be a useful way to measure your personal progress, and it's exciting and fun. Bring your family to cheer you on.

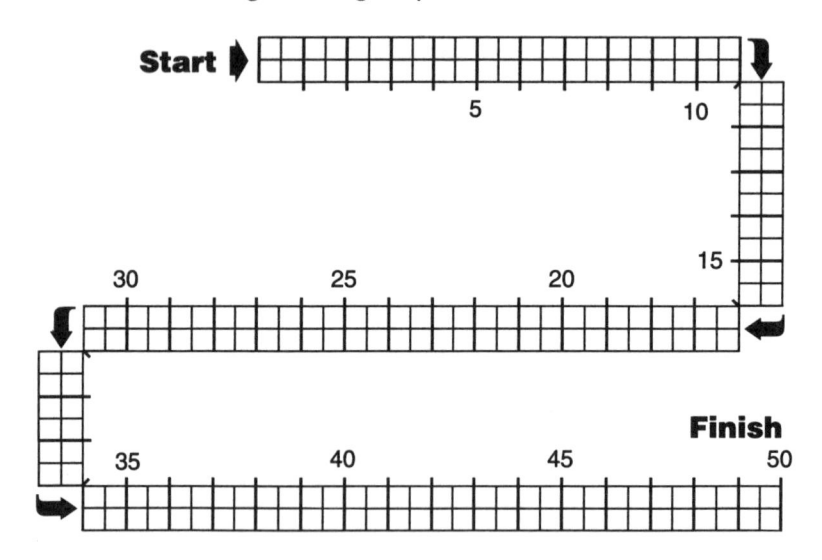

You can participate on a local, regional, national, and even international level. For more information, check your local Masters association. Use these sources to get more information:

U.S. Masters Swimming, Inc.
2 Peters Ave.
Rutland, MA 01543
508-886-6631

Swim Magazine/Sports Publishers
228 Nevada St.
El Segundo, CA 90245
310-607-9956

Masters Sports Magazine
400 E. 85th St., Ste. 9D
New York, NY 10028
212-535-7550

Synchronized Swimming

You might also consider joining an organized synchronized swimming group. You can participate in synchronized swimming solo or in a duet, trio, or group or team. Check your local YMCA, YWCA, or community center for groups, classes, clinics, demonstrations, competitions, and swim shows.

Those of you who may want a low-key competitive program should consider Masters Synchronized Swimming, a national program for those over age 19. For information about rules and how to reach your local associations, contact U.S. Synchronized Swimming, Inc., at (317) 237-5700.

Those of you interested in getting up-to-date information about synchronized swimming should try *Synchro*, which you can order from

Synchro Swimming USA
United States Synchronized Swimming
201 S. Capitol Ave., Ste. 501
Indianapolis, IN 46225

Water Play With Your Newborn

Swimming is the ideal family activity—fun and safe for all. One of the best gifts you can give a little one is to teach him or her how to safely enjoy the pleasures of swimming and water play. It's a gift your child will keep for life and that you will enjoy giving.

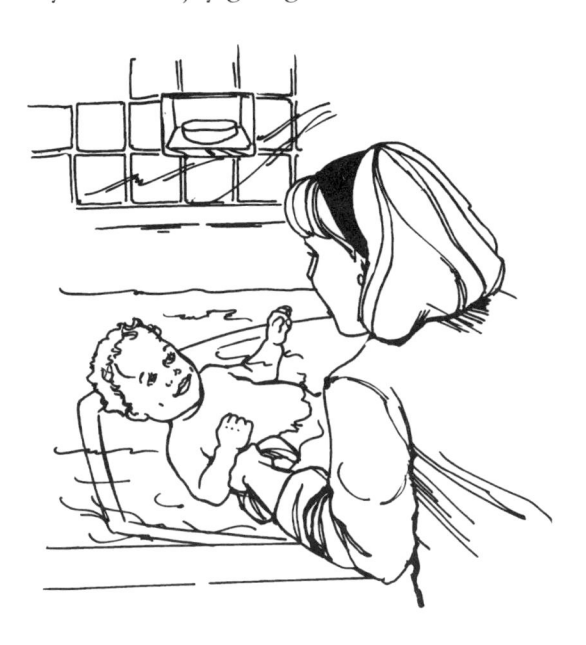

You can introduce your child to the joys of water almost immediately after birth. Remember, a water environment is familiar to your infant, as he has just spent 9 months in amniotic fluid. An infant in water instinctively paddles and holds her breath if she submerges (although she will lack the strength to get her face above the water to breathe).

It is very important to project a positive attitude when introducing your baby to water. Your baby will enjoy the water only if he senses that you are comfortable and confident in the water. Babies are very receptive to the emotions of people around them, and if your infant senses that you are afraid or uncomfortable, then she will tend to find experience in the water unpleasant and even frightening. Children *learn* to be afraid of the water; it is not an innate response.

If you bring your infant to the water using the proper approach, you'll be starting her on the road to a lifetime of safety, fun, and fitness. Water play helps develop your baby's muscular strength, coordination, and balance. There are even some indications that children who engage in water play and swimming at an early age are healthier, more intelligent, and more sociable than those who don't—a real plus for your child. And, of course, teaching your baby how to stay afloat will give him an important safety skill. In addition, a very special bond that can enhance your relationship forever develops as you work with your baby in the water.

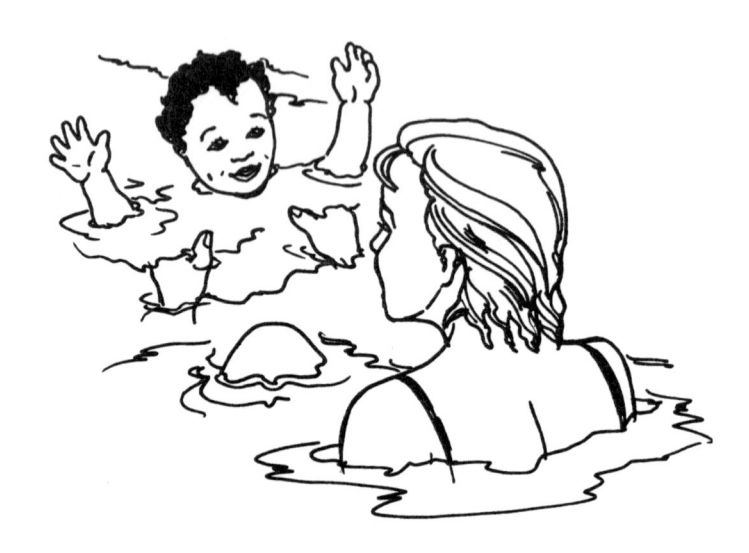

Naturally, you must use common sense with your baby in the water. You have to remember that your baby has no control over her world, and you should be careful to avoid the shock of temperature changes, sudden immersions, or rough water. You should also keep a close watch on your baby's health and the hygiene of the swimming facility. *Never, ever, leave your baby alone in or around water* or divert your attention from your baby even for a moment. Also keep your expectations reasonable—no 2-year-old is ready to swim the length of a pool. Few if any infants can swim alone for more than several seconds. A child usually is physically capable of sustained independent swimming only when he reaches 3 years old.

Before you take your baby to the pool you should know basic safety skills so that you are at ease in the water. You should also know CPR (cardiopulmonary resuscitation) and mouth-to-mouth resuscitation. Check for courses at your local American Red Cross chapter or American Heart Association.

If you use common sense and care, you and your baby will both have a rewarding experience in the water. And you may find that you will learn things about your baby and your relationship with her.

Family Swimming Programs

As your child grows, he will be able to master more of the basic swimming skills and to participate in a swimming program that will help him develop a fit and healthy body along with a love of the water.

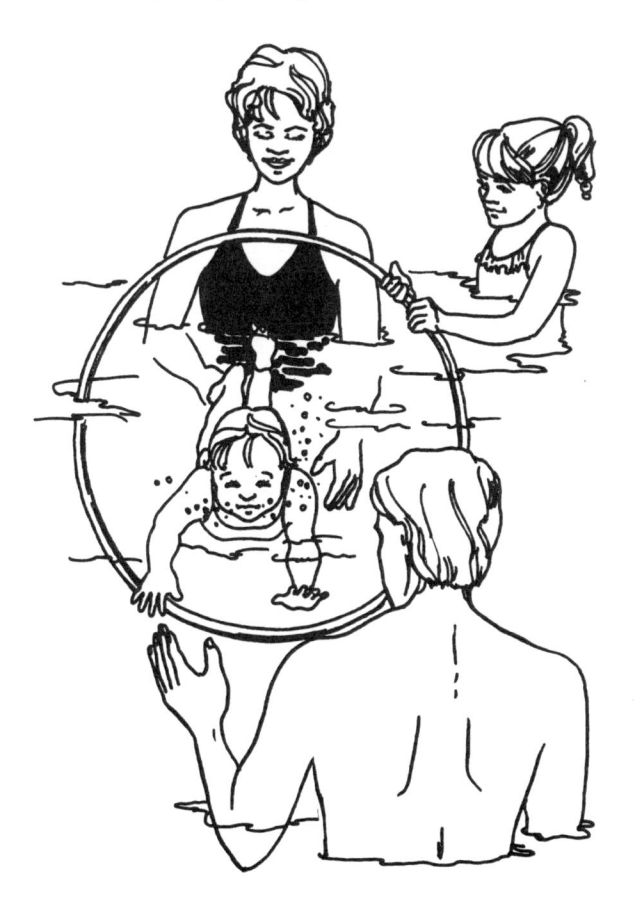

A preschool-age child is ready to be enrolled in an organized program where she can learn proper swimming techniques and water safety. Often the facilities used in these programs and classes have a raised platform in the pool that adjusts the pool depth to about 2 feet. Look for a preschool program run by an experienced staff that places priority on water safety. Swimming programs for children ages 3 to 5, if well designed, should be progressive in nature.

What swimming skills can you expect your child to learn at this age? Most children will be able to learn water-adjustment skills, breathing techniques, prone and supine floats, a basic crawl stroke, and how to change positions in the water from back to front and vice versa.

Several national organizations (a list follows) have information about places to find swimming facilities and programs for both children and adults. In addition, you can check your local Yellow Pages under the following headings: Municipal Department of Parks and Recreation, Schools, Community Centers, and Swim and Health Clubs.

> American Camping Association
> National Headquarters
> Bradford Woods
> 5000 State Road 67 North
> Martinsville, IN 46151-7902
> 317-342-8456

Serves as a national clearinghouse on information about aquatic resources in camping facilities.

> American Red Cross National Headquarters
> Corporate Communications-Public Inquiry
> 431 18th Street N.W.
> Washington, DC 20006
> 202-737-8300

Directs you to local chapters that provide aquatic information, programs, and materials.

> Boy Scouts of America
> National Headquarters
> 1325 W. Walnut Hill Ln.
> Irving, TX 75038
> 214-580-2000

> Boys and Girls Clubs of America
> 100 Edgewood Avenue, Suite 700
> Atlanta, GA 30303
> 404-527-7100

Girl Scouts of the U.S.A.
National Headquarters
420 Fifth Ave.
New York, NY 10018-2702
212-852-8000

Provide information on local aquatic programs.

International Swimming Hall of Fame
One Hall of Fame Drive
Fort Lauderdale, FL 33316
305-462-6536

Stages swim-a-thons for raising funds for equipment, and operates an aquatic museum for all to enjoy.

National Jewish Community Center Association
15 East 26th St.
New York, NY 10010
212-532-4949

Runs local aquatic programs at Jewish community centers throughout the United States.

National Park Service
Department of the Interior
Office of Public Inquiry (04/1013)
P.O. Box 37127
Washington, DC 20013-7127
202-208-4747

Maps and guides for regional National Park Service seashore and lakeshore facilities for aquatics, recreation, and lodging. Allow up to eight weeks for information to arrive.

National Spa and Pool Institute
2111 Eisenhower Ave., Ste. 500
Alexandria, VA 22314
703-838-0083

The national trade association for manufacturers; promotes health and safety aspects of swimming and compiles a directory of publications about the industry's products.

National Swim School Association
776 21st Ave. N.
St. Petersburg, FL 33704
813-896-7946

National organization of swim schools, focusing on children's classes. Includes the National Swim Teachers of America.

President's Council on Physical Fitness and Sports
701 Pennsylvania Ave., Ste. 250
Washington, DC 20201
202-272-3421

Sponsors fitness programs throughout country.

United States Swimming, Inc.
c/o USOC
One Olympic Plaza
Colorado Springs, CO 80909
719-578-4578

Provides information about local competitive swimming, diving, synchronized swimming, long-distance swimming, and water polo programs throughout the United States.

Young Men's Christian Association of the U.S.
101 N. Wacker Dr.
Chicago, IL 60606
312-977-0031

Sponsors local YMCA comprehensive and progressive aquatic programs.

Young Women's Christian Association
National Headquarters
726 Broadway
New York, NY 10003
212-614-2700

Sponsors local aquatic programs throughout the country.

It is very important that you be directly involved with your child's swimming program. Your encouragement will make a big difference in how well your child participates and enjoys the program. Make a point of swimming with your child outside of the class, keeping abreast of her accomplishments, and helping her master skills. Your child will enjoy the program more, and so will you. Remember, it's a family affair!

Appendix

This appendix contains two forms that may be helpful to your water fitness program. Feel free to photocopy them for easy use. The first is a personal workout log to help you keep track of your water fitness program. Fill in this log with the details of your workout—the date, how long you swam or exercised, and how you felt during your workout. It will be a guide that helps you determine what is comfortable and useful for yourself. The information you record in this log may also be useful to your doctor.

The second form will enable you to create your own water fitness workout, if you desire. You can use this to plan a series of exercises that you feel would comprise a good workout, or to record a workout that combines water exercises and lap swimming. This template helps you preserve the workout on paper. The template includes space for the warm-up, main set, and cool-down exercises. Don't forget to include a warm-up and cool-down in your workouts.

Personal Water Fitness Log

Date	Lap swim workout			Water exercise workout		Warm-up/cool-down time (minutes)	Total time	Comments
	Number	Distance	Time (min)	Number	Time (minutes)			

Create Your Own Workout

Personal focus _____   **Month** _____

Workout component	Water exercise or lap swim	Comments
Warm-up (5 minutes)	_____	_____
	_____	_____
	_____	_____
	_____	_____
	_____	_____
Main set /swim	_____	_____
Level 1 (10 minutes)	_____	_____
Level 2 (15 minutes)	_____	_____
Level 3 (20 minutes)	_____	_____
	_____	_____
	_____	_____
	_____	_____
	_____	_____
	_____	_____
	_____	_____
Cool-down (5 minutes)	_____	_____
	_____	_____
	_____	_____
	_____	_____

Workout notes: _____
_____
_____
_____
_____

INDEX

A

Abdominal exercises
  benefits of, 55, 65
  strengthening, 33, 55, 58-59, 60, 62, 65, 66, 72, 73
  stretching/flexibility, 55, 57, 68, 71
  warm-ups/cool-downs, 33
Adjusting to water, 28, 30
Alternate breathing, 92
Apple picking, 122
Aqua lunge, 35
Arm and leg reach, 76
Arm circle, 49
Arm exercises
  strengthening, 49, 53, 54
  stretching/flexibility, 76
Arm motion for swimming, elements of, 84
Arm press, 47-48

B

Back exercises
  benefits of, 55
  strengthening, 55, 58-59, 62, 66
  stretching/flexibility, 58-59, 66, 71
  warm-ups/cool-downs, 32, 33
Back extension, 58-59
Back flutter kick, 106, 108, 111, 114
Back massage, 63
Back pain/strain
  exercises for, 6, 55, 58-59, 62, 70, 80, 151
  swimming for, 111, 182
Backstroke
  elementary, 105-106
  practice exercises, 46, 113-114
  sculling, 103-105
  technique for, 103-112
  with water ballet, 179
  windmill, 106-108
Benefits of water exercise
  of breathing exercises, 37
  of exercises for specific parts of body, 45, 55, 65, 75
  overview of, 3, 5-7, 9-10
  of strengthening exercises, 5-6, 45, 55, 65
  of stretching/flexibility exercises, 6, 45, 55, 65
Bent-arm S-pull, 108
Bent-knee marching step, 184
Bicycle pedal, 67
Blood pressure, 6
Blood supply, 6
Body alignment, exercises for, 32, 33, 55, 80
Body position for swimming, defined, 84
Bradley childbirth technique, 8
Breaststroke
  practice exercises, 46, 99-101
  technique for, 95-98
  with water ballet, 179
Breaststroke arm pull, 99
Breathe and bob, 41
Breathe and reach, 39
Breathing, basic guidelines for, 17
Breathing, for swimming
  with backstroke, 104, 106, 108
  basic principles, 84
  with breaststroke, 96, 98
  with butterfly stroke, 186
  with crawl stroke, 86, 92, 93
  rhythmic breathing, 86, 93
  with sidestroke, 117
Breathing exercises
  basic guidelines, 37
  benefits of, 37
  breathe and bob, 41

225

Breathing exercises *(continued)*
  breathe and reach, 39
  breathing with head circles, 40
  cleansing breath, 17, 38
  for crawl stroke, 93
  effleurage with, 17, 36
  labor/delivery breathing
    patterns, 42-43
  rhythmic breathing, 93
Breathing with head circles, 40
Buoyancy, 9, 83
Butterfly stroke
  practice exercises, 191-192
  safety guidelines, 14
  technique for, 186-190
Buttocks, exercises for, 71

C
Calf exercises, 29, 69
Calf stretch, 69
Caps, 18
Cardiorespiratory fitness, 3
Catch, definition of, 84
Catch-up arm stroke, 94
Center of gravity
  exercising and, 55
  swimming and, 83-84
Charley horse, exercise for
  avoiding, 65
Chest exercises, 53, 54
Children, swimming for, 215-220
Chloasma, 14
Chlorine, effects of, 14
Circle spray, 56
Circulatory system, 7
Clam, 181
Cleansing breath, 17, 38
Clocks, 17, 20
Concentration, exercises for, 58-59
Conditioning, exercises for, 75, 78, 81-82
Cool-downs and warm-ups. *See* Warm-ups and cool-downs
Coordination, exercises for, 75, 81-82

Crawl stroke
  practice exercises, 46, 93-94
  technique for, 85-92
  trudgen crawl, 119
  with water ballet, 179
Crossover kick, 88

D
Deep-water jog, 81-82
Deep water workouts, summarized, 4
Delivery, exercises during, 17, 36
Delivery, exercises for preparation for
  benefits of, 55, 65
  breathing, 37-43
  strengthening, 55
  stretching/flexibility, 65
  warm-ups/cool-downs, 34
Delivery, methods for. *See* Prepared childbirth
Delivery breathing patterns, 42-43
Diet, 15, 16
Distances, guidelines for judging, 126
Diving, prohibition of, 89
Dolphin kick, 186, 188-191
Dolphin sit and kick, 191
Double leg circle, 73

E
Edema, 10, 65
Effleurage, 17, 36
Elementary backstroke, 105-106
Equipment, 17-21
Exercise workouts
  basic guidelines, 10-11, 13-17, 25-26, 123-127
  month 2, 130-132
  month 3, 135-136
  month 4, 142-143
  month 5, 146-148
  month 6, 151-153

month 7, 158-160
month 8, 164-166
month 9, 169-171
overview of, 4
when to use, 123-124

F
Family swimming programs, 217-220
Feet flex, 29
Fins
   description of, 18
   exercises with, 76
First-trimester workouts
   basic guidelines, 10-11, 13-17, 129-130
   month 2 exercise workouts, 130-132
   month 2 swim workouts, 132-134
   month 3 exercise workouts, 135-136
   month 3 swim workouts, 137-139
Flexibility exercises. *See* Stretching and flexibility exercises
Flip turns, prohibition of, 90
Flotation supports
   description of, 20
   exercises with, 34, 78, 81
Fluid replacement, 16
Flutterfly stroke, 190
Flutter kick (exercise), 66
Flutter kick, with strokes, 86, 106, 108, 111, 114
Frog kick, 96, 98, 100-101

G
Goggles, 18

H
Hand paddles
   description of, 18
   exercises with, 47-50, 52
Hang 10, 51

Head circles, breathing with, 40
Heart rate monitoring, 16
Heat illness, 11, 14
Hemorrhoids, 34
Hip exercises
   strengthening, 60
   stretching/flexibility, 61, 62, 71
Hip touch, 57
Hot tubs, 11
Hyperinsulinemia, 16

I
Infants, water play with, 215-217
Interval training, 138
Inverted scissors kick, 117

J
Jacuzzi baths, 11, 14
Jog, deep-water, 81-82
Jumping, prohibition of, 89

K
Kegel exercises, 34, 178
Kickboard press, 54
Kickboards, description of, 18
Kicks, with swimming strokes
   with backstroke, 104, 106, 108, 111, 114
   with breaststroke, 96, 98, 100-101
   with butterfly stroke, 186, 188-191
   with crawl stroke, 86, 88, 92
   crossover kick, 88
   dolphin kick, 186, 188-191
   flutter kick, 86, 106, 108, 111, 114
   frog kick, 96, 98, 100-101
   scissors kick, 117
   with sidestroke, 117, 119
   whip kick, 96, 98
Knee lift, wall, 62

L
Labor, exercises for preparation for
   benefits of, 55

Labor, exercises *(continued)*
  breathing, 37-43
  effleurage, 17, 36
  strengthening, 55
Labor and delivery breathing patterns (exercise), 42-43
Lamaze childbirth technique
  description of, 7-8
  instructions for exercises for, 36-43
Leboyer childbirth technique, 7
Leg circle, double, 73
Leg exercises. *See also* Calf exercises; Thigh exercises
  strengthening, 66, 72
  stretching/flexibility, 61, 66, 68, 70, 71, 76
Leg lift, 71
Leg motion for swimming, elements of, 84. *See also* Kicks, with swimming strokes
Leg scissors, 68
Leg swirl, 72
Log, sample form, 222
Lower-back pain
  exercises for, 55, 58-59, 62, 151
  swimming for, 111, 182
Lower-body exercises
  benefits of, 65
  bicycle pedal, 67
  calf stretch, 69
  double leg circle, 73
  feet flex, 29
  flutter kick, 66
  leg lift, 71
  leg scissors, 68
  leg swirl, 72
  strengthening, 65, 66, 69, 72, 73
  stretching/flexibility, 29, 35, 61, 65, 68, 69, 70, 71, 73, 76
  swing and sway, 61
  wall walk, 70

M

Main set, basic guidelines for, 25-26, 124
Marlin turn, 181
Massage, 63
Masters swimming, 213-214
Medley of pulls, 46
Melasma, 14
Middle-body exercises
  back extension, 58-59
  back massage, 63
  benefits of, 55
  circle spray, 56
  hip touch, 57
  pelvic tilt, 33
  sit-up, modified, 60
  strengthening, 33, 55, 58, 60, 62
  stretching/flexibility, 55, 56, 57, 58, 61, 62
  swing and sway, 61
  wall knee lift, 62
Modified sit-up, 60

N

Natural childbirth, 7. *See also* Prepared childbirth
Neck exercises, 40, 51, 52
Newborns, water play with, 215-217
Nutrition, 15, 16

O

Overhead stretch, 27
Overheating, 11, 14, 16

P

Pace clocks, 17, 20
Paddles. *See* Hand paddles
Pelvic floor exercises, 34, 65
Pelvic girdle, 5
Pelvic tilt, 33
Pendulum body swing, 77
Perineal exercises, 34
Personal water fitness log, sample form, 222

Postpartum workouts
　basic guidelines, 15-16, 177-178
　butterfly stroke in, 186-190
　water ballet in, 178-185
　week 1 swim workout, 193-194
　week 2 swim workout, 194-195
　week 3 swim workout, 196-197
　week 4 swim workout, 198-199
　week 5 swim workout, 199-200
　week 6 swim workout, 201-202
　week 7 swim workout, 203-205
　week 8 swim workout, 205-207
　week 9 swim workout, 207-208
　week 10 swim workout, 208-209
　week 11 swim workout, 210-211
　week 12 swim workout, 211-212
Posture, exercises for, 32, 33, 55, 80
Posture check, 80
Prepared childbirth
　description of methods for, 7-8
　instructions for exercises for, 17, 36-43
Presses
　arm press, 47-48
　kickboard press, 54
Pull, definition of, 84
Pull-buoys, 18
Pulls, medley of, 46
Push-off
　with backstroke, 108, 110
　with breaststroke, 98
　with butterfly stroke, 187
　with crawl stroke, 89-90
　with sidestroke, 118
Push-ups, 53

R
Recovery, in swimming strokes, 84
Relaxation exercises, 36, 63
Rhythmic breathing, with crawl stroke, 86, 93
Rope jump, 192

S
Safety guidelines
　for infant/toddler water play, 216-217
　for water workouts, 10-11, 13-15, 126-127
Saunas, 11, 14
Scissors kick, 117
Scull and hug, 113
Sculling
　backstroke, 103-105
　with water ballet, 180
Sculling (exercise), 52
Second-trimester workouts
　basic guidelines, 10-11, 13-17, 141
　month 4 exercise workouts, 142-143
　month 4 swim workouts, 144-146
　month 5 exercise workouts, 146-148
　month 5 swim workouts, 148-151
　month 6 exercise workouts, 151-153
　month 6 swim workouts, 153-156
Shark circle, 185
Shoes, 20
Shoulder exercises
　strengthening, 49, 53, 54

Shoulder exercises *(continued)*
  stretching/flexibility, 31
Shoulder shrug, 31
Side muscle stretches, 77, 119
Sidestroke
  practice exercises, 46, 120-122
  technique for, 115-122
  with water ballet, 179
Sit and kick, 28, 191
Sit-up, modified, 60
Sport swing, 50
S-shaped pull
  with backstroke, 108
  with crawl stroke, 88, 94
Stand tall, 32
Steam rooms, 11
Strengthening exercises
  for abdomen, 33, 55, 58-59, 60, 62, 65, 66, 72, 73
  for arms, 49, 53, 54
  for back, 55, 58-59, 62, 66
  benefits of, 5-6, 45, 55, 65
  for calves, 69
  for chest, 53, 54
  for hips, 60
  for legs in general, 66, 72
  lower-body, 65, 66, 69, 72, 73
  middle-body, 33, 55, 58, 60, 62
  for perineal muscles, 34
  for shoulders, 49, 53, 54
  for thighs, 58-59, 60
  upper-body, 46, 47-48, 49, 50, 53, 54
  warm-ups/cool-downs, 33, 34
Stretching and flexibility exercises
  for abdomen, 55, 57, 68, 71
  for arms, 76
  for back, 58-59, 66, 71
  basic guidelines, 17, 25, 26
  benefits of, 6, 45, 55, 65
  with breathing exercises, 40
  for buttocks, 71
  for calves, 29, 69
  for hips, 61, 62, 71
  for legs in general, 61, 66, 68, 70, 71, 76
  lower-body, 29, 35, 61, 65, 68, 69, 70, 71, 73, 76
  middle-body, 55, 56, 57, 58, 61, 62
  for neck, 40, 51, 52
  for shoulders, 31
  for side muscles, 77, 119
  for thighs, 35, 65, 68, 70, 73
  upper-body, 31, 40, 45, 47-48, 51
  warm-ups/cool-downs, 25, 26, 27, 29, 31, 35
Stroke coordination, 84
Stroke count, defined, 137
Strokes. *See also* Backstroke; Breaststroke; Butterfly stroke; Crawl stroke; Sidestroke
  basic principles for, 83-84
  elementary backstroke, 105-106
  flutterfly, 190
  practice exercises, 46, 93-94, 99-101, 113-114, 120-122
  sculling, 103-105
  trudgen crawl, 119
  with water ballet, 179-180
  windmill backstroke, 106-108
Sun, protection from, 14
Swim fins. *See* Fins
Swimming, for infants and children, 215-220
Swimming, Masters, 213-214
Swimming, synchronized, 215
Swimming caps, 18
Swimming workouts. *See also* Postpartum workouts
  basic guidelines, 10-11, 13-17, 123-127
  month 2, 132-134
  month 3, 137-139
  month 4, 144-146
  month 5, 148-151

month 6, 153-156
month 7, 161-164
month 8, 166-169
month 9, 171-173
Swim strokes. *See* Strokes
Swimsuits, 17-18
Swing and sway, 61
Synchronized swimming, 215

T
Temperature, of body, 11, 14, 16
Temperature, of water, 11, 13
Thigh exercises
   benefits of, 65
   strengthening, 58-59, 60
   stretching/flexibility, 35, 65, 68, 70, 73
Third-trimester workouts
   basic guidelines, 10-11, 13-17, 157-158
   month 7 exercise workouts, 158-160
   month 7 swim workouts, 161-164
   month 8 exercise workouts, 164-166
   month 8 swim workouts, 166-169
   month 9 exercise workouts, 169-171
   month 9 swim workouts, 171-173
Toddlers, water play with, 216-217
Total body exercises
   arm and leg reach, 76
   benefits of, 75
   deep-water jog, 81-82
   pendulum body swing, 77
   posture check, 80
   treading, 78-79
Treading, 78-79
Trudgen crawl, 119
Tuck turn, 182
Turns
   with backstroke, 110
   with breaststroke, 98
   with butterfly stroke, 190
   with crawl stroke, 90-91
   marlin turn, 181
   with sidestroke, 118-119
   tuck turn, 182
   with water ballet, 181-182

U
Under and over, 120
Upper-body exercises
   arm circle, 49
   arm press, 47-48
   benefits of, 45
   hang 10, 51
   kickboard press, 54
   medley of pulls, 46
   sculling, 52
   shoulder shrug, 31
   sport swing, 50
   strengthening, 46, 47-48, 49, 50, 53, 54
   stretching/flexibility, 31, 40, 45, 47-48, 51
   wall push-up, 53
Uterus, 5

V
Varicose veins, 6, 65

W
Walk/jog, water, 30
Wall knee lift, 62
Wall push-up, 53
Wall walk, 70
Warm-ups and cool-downs
   for adjusting to water, 28, 30
   aqua lunge, 35
   for back muscles, 32, 33
   basic guidelines, 16, 25-26, 124
   for body alignment, 32, 33
   definition of, 25, 26
   effleurage, 17, 36

Warm-ups and cool-downs *(continued)*
  feet flex, 29
  overhead stretch, 27
  pelvic tilt, 33
  for preparing for labor/delivery, 34, 36
  shoulder shrug, 31
  sit and kick, 28
  stand tall, 32
  strengthening, 33, 34
  stretching/flexibility, 25, 26, 27, 29, 31, 35
  water Kegel, 34, 178
  water walk/jog, 30
Watches, 17, 18
Water ballet exercises
  basic guidelines, 178-180
  bent-knee marching step, 184
  clam, 183
  marlin turn, 181
  shark circle, 185
  tuck turn, 182
Water birth, 8
Water exercise, definition of, 4
Water Kegel, 34, 178
Water play with infants and toddlers, 215-217
Water shoes, 20
Water walk/jog, 30
Weight control, 7, 10
Whip kick, 96, 98
Windmill backstroke, 106-108
Workouts. *See also* Exercise workouts; First-trimester workouts; Postpartum workouts; Second-trimester workouts; Swimming workouts; Third-trimester workouts
  basic guidelines, 10-11, 15-17, 123-127
  sample form for creating, 223

ABOUT THE AUTHOR

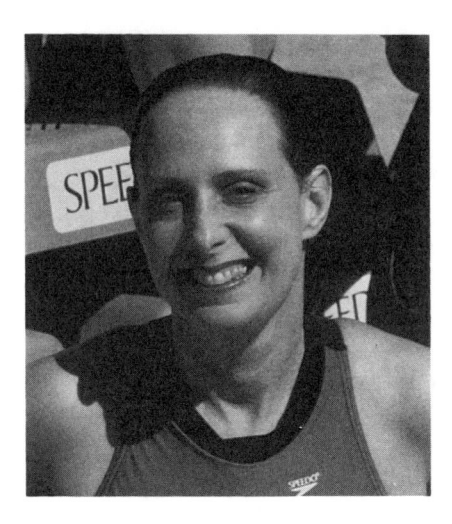

Dr. Jane Katz, EdD, has been a pioneer in water exercise and physical fitness, working in the aquatics field for more than 30 years. She has been a member of the U.S. Masters All-American swimming, long distance, and synchronized Swimming Teams since 1974 and continues to win world championships. As a professor of health, physical education, and athletics at the City University of New York, Dr. Katz has taught swimming, water exercise, and fitness to thousands of people and lectured at clinics worldwide. For more than 15 years she has studied and seen first-hand how water fitness benefits pregnant women.

Dr. Katz received her doctorate from Columbia University, where she specialized in leisure studies and gerontology. Since then she has made numerous television appearances and written hundreds of magazine articles on aquatic fitness and water exercise. She is the author of five previous books, including *Swimming for Total Fitness, The W.E.T. Workout®, Swim 30 Laps in 30 Days, FitnessWorks!™*, and *Swimming Through Your Pregnancy*.

Dr. Katz is a trustee member of the National Council on Women's Health and has been a consultant to the President's Council on Physical Fitness and Sports and a member of the board of directors of the National Fitness Leaders Association. She was appointed by the International Swimming Hall of Fame to serve on its international congress board and is an advisory board member of several organizations, including the Aquatic Exercise Association, the U.S. Water Fitness Association, and *Aquatics International*. She has been a water safety instructor trainer for the Red Cross of America for over 30 years.

— More great exercise books from — Human Kinetics

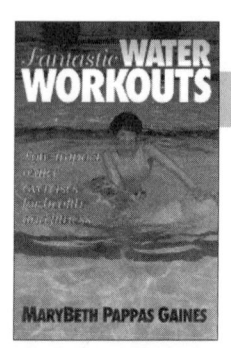

Fantastic Water Workouts

MaryBeth Pappas Gaines
1993 • Paper • 184 pp
Item PGAI0458 • ISBN 0-87322-458-2
$14.95 ($19.95 Canadian)

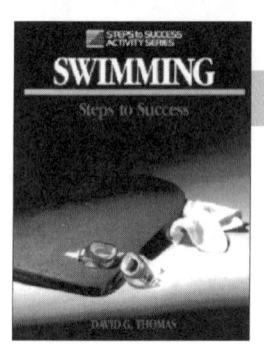

Swimming

Steps to Success
David G. Thomas, MS
1989 • Paper • 192 pp
Item PTHO0309 • ISBN 0-88011-309-X
$14.95 ($19.95 Canadian)

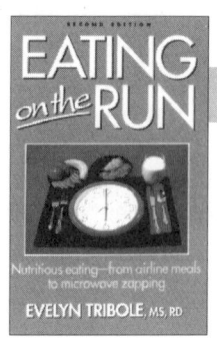

Eating on the Run

Second Edition
Evelyn Tribole, MS, RD
1992 • Paper • 256 pp
Item PTRI0452 • ISBN 0-88011-452-5
$14.95 ($19.95 Canadian)

Place your order using the appropriate telephone number/address shown in the front of this book, or **call toll-free in the U.S. (1-800-747-4457)**.

Prices subject to change.

Human Kinetics